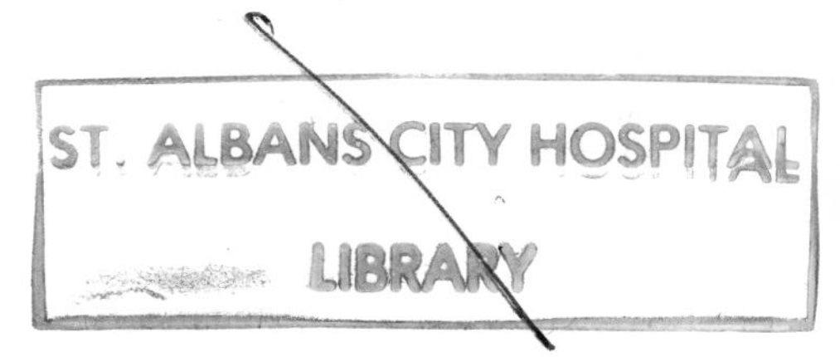

Environmental & Occupational risks *of health care*

British Medical Association

June 1994

Environmental and Occupational Risks of Health Care

A publication from the BMA Scientific Affairs Department

Chairman, Board of Science and Education:	Professor Jack Howell
Head, BMA Ethics, Science and Information Divison:	Dr Fleur Fisher
Editor:	David R Morgan
Consultant Writer:	Dr Jeremy Beach
Contributors:	Mike Arrowsmith Dr Chris Collins Professor Anthony Dayan Dr William Dixon Hilary Glanville Erica Ison Tony Jones Graham Jukes Dr Brian Keeble Dr Gordon Macpherson Sarah Mars Sallie Robins Mr W M Ross Dr Chris Stenton
Editorial Secretariat:	Hayley Todd
Indexer:	Richard Jones
Design:	Hilary Glanville

British Library Cataloguing-in-Publication Data
A catalogue record for this book is available from the British Library

ISBN 0 7279 0887 1

First published in 1994 by: British Medical Association, Tavistock Square, London WC1H 9JP

Printed by: The Chameleon Press, London

Acknowledgement

Thanks are due to the following copyright owners for permission to reproduce their photographs:

The National Radiological Protection Board
The BMA Archive
Colemans of Norwich Archives
The Viral Hepatitis Prevention Board

The Association is particularly grateful to The Wellcome Centre/National Medical Slide Bank for their help and support in illustrating this publication.

Contents

Abbreviations and acronyms

AIDS	Acquired immunodeficiency syndrome
ALARA	as low as reasonably achievable
BATNEEC	best available technique not entailing excessive cost
BMA	British Medical Association
BS	British Standard
CCDC	Consultant in Communicable Disease Control
COSHH	Control of Substances Hazardous to Health Regulations (1988)
CT	computed tomography
DHA	District Health Authority
DNA	Deoxyribonucleic acid
ECETOC	European Chemical Industry Ecology & Toxicology Centre
FHSA	Family Health Service Authority
FOM	Faculty of Occupational Medicine
HBV	Hepatitis B virus
HCV	Hepatitis C virus
HIV	Human immunodeficiency virus
HSC	Health and Safety Commission
HSWA	Health and Safety at Work etc Act (1974)
IARC	International Agency for Research on Cancer
ICRP	International Commission on Radiological Protection
IOH	Institute of Occupational Hygiene
ILO	International Labour Organisation
keV	kilo electron volts
KHz	kilohertz
l	litres
MeV	mega electron volts
MHz	megahertz
ml	mililitres
ManSv	man Sieverts

mSv	milli Sieverts
NHS	National Health Service
NHSE	National Health Service Executive
NRPB	National Radiological Protection Board
OES	Occupational Exposure Standard
ppm	parts per million
RBE	relative biological effectiveness
RHA	Regional Health Authority
RIDDOR	Reporting of Injuries, Diseases and Dangerous Occurrences Regulations (1985)
UK	United Kingdom
UNSCEAR	United Nations Scientific Committee on the Effects of Atomic Radiation
μSv	micro Sieverts
VDU	visual display unit
WHO	World Health Organisation

List of tables and figures

Tables

Figures

Introduction

Health care is a diverse 'industry' comprising many different workers in a range of working environments. These include hospitals, clinics, laboratories, nursing homes, workshops, patients' homes and factories, containing much modern technology aimed at making ill people well, or keeping well people healthy. These objectives generate great commercial and moral pressures for the development of new technology. Any new discovery promising to achieve these objectives can arouse public interest, and although much health care is routine, some, such as treatments for cancer, are publicly emotive issues. There is often great pressure to maximise potential benefits to patients in a short time, perhaps before a full risk assessment of the environmental impact of a new technology or process has been possible.

This report sets out for both general and professional readers existing evidence relating to the environmental and occupational risks arising from medical practice. Risks arising from health care can be broadly divided into three groups; those arising within the workplace to employees, those affecting patients — the consumers of health care — and those arising in the wider environment to the general population. Risks may arise from handling novel drugs and chemicals, from exposure to radiation used for new diagnostic and therapeutic applications, from contact with infectious agents, and from numerous other processes which are carried out in the health care environment. This report does not, however, address the clinical implications of treatment, as these are covered extensively in the medical literature. Risks facing employees and patients may extend beyond the place where they are generated and so may present a risk to the general public, and the wider environment; an environment that may stretch for many hundreds of miles, and may encompass many biological species.

Health care workers have customarily put the interests of patients before their own welfare. Until recently, the NHS enjoyed Crown immunity from prosecution if it contravened the regulations on health and safety that applied to industry and commerce. The removal of Crown immunity and an increasing awareness of the importance of occupational health among employees, as well as society's environmental concerns are beginning to redress this balance somewhat, forcing those providing health care to consider more carefully the implications of their actions. Recent health and safety and environmental legislation have introduced the fundamental concept of risk assessment as an essential first step in managing and reducing risk.

As well as its duty to employees, the health care industry has responsibilities and a 'duty of care' for the environment, particularly in relation to waste disposal. It should also act in a responsible way to society as a whole, leading by example, to ensure that there are no adverse environmental consequences as a result of its activities. Indeed, the NHS Estates Management acknowledged this duty in 1992 in the following statement, "...it is particularly appropriate that the NHS should adopt pro-environmental policies. The NHS is in the business of health care and its promotion, and a healthier environment means a healthier population. It is not acceptable for the NHS to despoil the environment and thus risk an increase in general ill health."[1]

Consideration of environmental factors associated with health care will be important in taking forward the programme of sustainable development which was one of the four main products of the United Nations Conference on Environment and Development (Earth Summit) which was held in Rio de Janeiro in 1992.[2] However, the United Nations Environment and Development Committee for the UK has commented that the report of the Government's strategy on sustainable development published in January 1994 fails to address major issues concerning the importance of the relationship between the environment and health.

BMA policy on the environment

During the past few years the British Medical Association (BMA) has produced a number of policy documents which consider environmental health and pollution and which contain policies for national action by government and by other organisations and individuals, with specific recommendations affecting the medical and allied professions. In addition, the BMA has been concerned about standards of health and safety in medical practice, particularly in the National Health Service (NHS). Most recently, it has researched and published a number of reports covering occupational health, and the environment — subjects of increasing scientific and public concern. The advent of the Acquired Immune Deficiency Syndrome (AIDS) epidemic in the United Kingdom (UK), led the Association to review procedures used in hospitals and in primary health care, to prevent cross-infection. The Association's reports on hepatitis and Human Immunodeficiency Syndrome (HIV), infection control in general practice, and the safe use and disposal of sharps were published and are used for training throughout the health care sector and in UK medical schools.[3,4]

In 1991 the BMA published *Hazardous Waste and Human Health,*[5] a comprehensive guide to a subject receiving much public and media attention. This was followed in January 1992 by *Pesticides, Chemicals and Health,*[6] a report that examined the risks to human health from acute and chronic exposure to chemicals in the environment. Also in 1992, the BMA's report *Cycling Towards Health and Safety*[7] considered the benefits to health and the environment, which would stem from an increase in cycling in the UK. The report concluded that a decrease in the number and speed of motor vehicles would lead to a reduction in the degree of injuries sustained by cyclists and pedestrians, and a reduction in environmental pollution caused by carbon monoxide, nitrogen dioxide, particulate hydrocarbon and carcinogens such as benzene.

The medical profession has a major role to play in exploring risks to human health so that hazards can be controlled or eliminated. The practical recommendations that arose from the BMA's work on the environment called for doctors to, "set an example of responsible waste management" and urged them to take part in, "managing the environment in the interests of public health". This further report from the BMA is aimed at continuing the debate and raising environmental and occupational health issues associated with health care. It represents the next logical step, with doctors looking at how to put their own house — the health care sector — in order.

In 1990 doctors at the Annual Representative Meeting of the British Medical Association called for the association to consider the specific effects of modern medical technology on the environment. Responding to this decision, in October 1991, the BMA's Board of Science and Education launched a study of the physical, social and psychological risks to health care workers, patients and the general public resulting from the use of medical practices and technology. This report aims to identify the potential hazards arising from health care and form a strategy for their control. The report primarily relates to those who work in the health services, and will also be of interest to students of medicine, nursing, environmental sciences and those interested in risk management and health and safety law and practice. Managers in the NHS and independent contractors will find this book a helpful guide to good practice and it should provide their staff with a wealth of information, to help ensure that the health care services are well managed and that resources are used safely and efficiently.

Scope of the report

Chapter 1 takes a brief look at the history of medical innovation and discovery over the last two centuries. It investigates the difficulties, hazards and benefits of introducing new practices.

Chapters 2, 3 and 4 address chemical hazards. Chapter 2 explains the functions and processes of environmental toxicology, and serves as a general background to the chapters that follow. Chapter 3 considers the proliferation of chemicals used in the health care industry and examines several potential problem substances. It reviews the evidence for potential adverse health effects among those exposed in the workplace. Chapter 4 deals with the use of anaesthetic gases and considers whether they pose any health risk to health care workers and the environment. Chapter 5 considers the physical hazard of radiation. It looks at health risks to the general public and health care workers from the medical use of radiation, and outlines the regulations and guidelines which control their use.

Chapters 6, 7 and 8 examine biological hazards. Chapter 6 explores routes of infection within the health care environment and strategies for managing these risks. The infection risks of viral hepatitis, HIV and tuberculosis are reviewed in detail. Chapter 7 analyses the risk presented to health care workers, the public and the environment by clinical waste from its point of generation, to the site of final disposal. It outlines a strategy for improving current practice. Chapter 8 investigates the rapidly changing field of genetic modification and its medical application. It looks into the systems which currently control these techniques and the prospects for their change.

Chapters 9, 10 and 11 address health, safety and environmental management. Chapter 9 discusses the current roles of occupational and public health medicine in protecting individuals from the adverse effects of health care. The prospects for developing these roles to meet the challenges of advancing health care are considered. Chapter 10 considers some of the themes discussed elsewhere in the report and examines how they relate to general medical practice, including health and safety, infection control and clinical waste. Chapter 11 explores some of the problems which arise from poor building design and maintenance and considers environmental management systems and the application of British Standard 7750 and staff retraining in this area. Chapter 12 presents the report's main findings and highlights the association's prime concerns. Recommendations are made requiring action at both national and local levels to control the environmental and occupational risks of health care.

This report was prepared under the auspices of the Board of Science and Education of the British Medical Association. The members of the Board in January 1994 were as follows:

Dr J L T Birley	(President, BMA)
Dr W J Appleyard	(Chairman, BMA Representative Body)
Dr A W Macara	(Chairman BMA Council)
Dr J A Riddell	(Treasurer, BMA)
Prof J B L Howell	(Chairman, BMA Board of Science and Education)
Dr L P Grime	(Deputy Chairman, BMA Board of Science and Education)
Dr J M Cundy	
Dr A Elliot	
Dr R Farrow	
Miss C E Fozzard	
Dr R Gilbert	
Dr A Mitchell	
Dr G M Mitchell	
Dr P Steadman	
Dr A Stewart	
Dr D Ward	

The members of the Working Party on Environmental and Occupational Risks of Health Care were as follows:

Sir Christopher Booth (Chairman)	Past Chairman, BMA Board of Science and Education, and Harvarian Librarian, Royal College of Physicians
Professor A D Dayan	Professor of Toxicology, St Bartholomew's Hospital Medical College, London
Dr W M Dixon	Past Chairman, BMA Occupational Health Committee, Occupational Health Consultant
Dr B R Keeble	Director of Public Health, Isle of Wight District Health Authority
Mr W M Ross	Past President, Royal College of Radiologists
Dr M J G Thomas	Past Member, Board of Science and Education

The Association is grateful for the specialist help provided by BMA Committees and many outside experts and organisations, and is particularly indebted to:

Mr Mike Arrowsmith,Chief Engineer, NHS Estates, Department of Health; Dr Peter Baxter, Consultant Occupational Physician, University of Cambridge; Dr Jeremy Beach, Clinical Lecturer, Institute of Occupational Health, University of Birmingham; Dr David Coggon, Reader in Occupational and Environmental Medicine, Medical Research Council Environmental Epidemiology Unit, Southampton; Dr Chris Collins, Retired Public Health Bacteriologist; Dr David Gompertz, Institute of Occupational Health, University of Birmingham; Mr Peter Hoffman, Laboratory of Hospital Infection, Central Public Health Laboratory; Mr Graham Jukes, Director, Professional and Technical Services, Institution of Environmental Health Officers; Mr Tony Jones, Senior Architect, NHS Estates, Department of Health; Dr Stella Lowry, Head of International Affairs, BMA; Dr Gordon Macpherson, former deputy editor, British Medical Journal; Dr Chris Stenton, Senior Lecturer in Occupational Medicine, Chest Unit and Regional Unit for Occupational Lung Disease, Newcastle General Hospital.

CHAPTER 1

Hazards of medical science

The past few decades have seen big advances in many technologies, including power generation, engineering, and information systems. Such advances have sometimes been achieved at a cost to the environment and the natural world. The pressure of an increasing population consuming ever greater amounts of energy, services, and manufactured goods during the 20th century are all too evident, and many people, realising past errors, are worried about the possible consequences. Destruction of rainforests and the ozone layer, pollution of water sources, the production of acid rain, photo-chemical smog, and the 'greenhouse effect', are well known examples, although controversy continues, over their exact causes and effects.

Scientific discovery

The exploitation of scientific discoveries and their incorporation into everyday life is occurring rapidly. Since the 19th century, improved technology and social and medical intervention in the lives of ordinary people have brought about striking improvements in health and quality of life. Towards the end of the century, the incidence of water and food-borne infectious diseases declined as a result of a series of public health measures, including such innovations as sanitation, the provision of clean water supplies, and the increasing regulation of food and drink.[1] But progress in medicine is rarely a smooth upward slope; it rather resembles an uneven staircase of changing and unpredictable challenges. As discoveries are made, medical practitioners must be convinced of their worth, but when innovations are introduced, they often bring fresh problems which may have adverse effects not only for the patient but also for health care staff and the environment.

However, some of the greatest innovations in health care over the past two centuries were not always recognised as the landmarks they later proved to be. A great challenge for the pioneer has been the task of convincing a sceptical profession of the importance of a discovery. At the other extreme, discoveries which arouse too much enthusiasm have also proved dangerous. The monument at the Röntgen Institute near Hamburg testifies to the enthusiastic welcome given to the discovery of x-rays. Among the early radiologists named on its stones are those who tragically assumed that the imperceptible radiation was harmless.

Antisepsis and asepsis

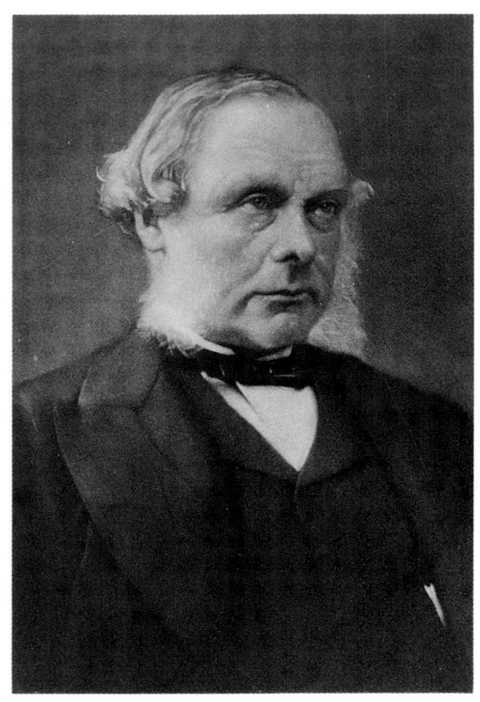

Joseph Lister, 1882

In Britain throughout the 19th and early part of the 20th centuries, infectious disease was the most important cause of death among all age groups and infant mortality was high. Hospitals and sanatoria were not free from such dangers and serious, even fatal, infections acquired by patients in the course of medical treatment were common. Deaths were particularly high among women in childbirth. In the Vienna of 1861, Ignaz Philipp Semmelweiss published his ideas on the spread of infection by doctors from the autopsy room to women in obstetric wards in, *The Cause, Concept, and Prophylaxis of Puerperal Fever* (quoted by Rhodes).[2] This aroused a storm of controversy but at the time gained limited acceptance.

The BMA was founded in 1832 "to promote the medical and allied sciences and maintain the honour and interests of the medical profession". It played a small part in the acceptance of the principles of antisepsis when Joseph Lister gave one of his earliest descriptions of his carbolic spray at a BMA Scientific Meeting in Plymouth in 1871. He is said to have convinced some of the more sceptical members of the audience by pointing to the dust suspended in a beam of sunlight as the cause of putrefaction. However, not everyone was convinced, *The Lancet* reported Lister's address in scathing terms. A leading article ran, "disbelievers in the marvellous efficacy of carbolic acid could not fail to notice that with every public appearance Professor Lister's solutions become weaker and weaker, while his faith

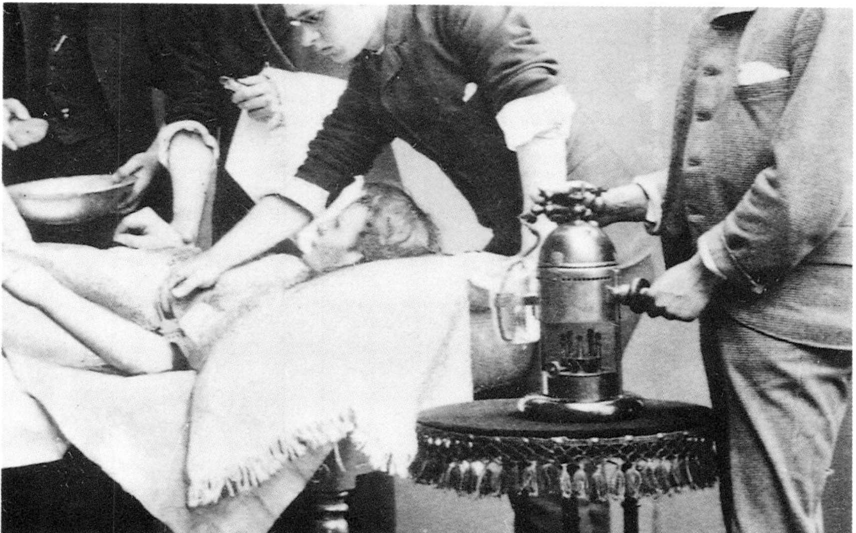

Surgical operation using carbolic spray , Aberdeen Royal Infirmary, circa 1880

appears to grow more and more."[3] Through this deep scepticism many lives were needlessly lost as doctors and nurses failed to be convinced of the importance of antisepsis.

The need for aseptic conditions grew more urgent as the potential for surgery expanded with the discovery of anaesthetic agents. Unlike the introduction of antisepsis, the benefits of the analgesic properties of nitrous oxide were easily demonstrable, gaining widespread recognition and leading to its use during many forms of surgery from the 1840s onwards.

Anaesthetic hazards

The benefits of anaesthesia were first recognised around 1800, when Sir Humphrey Davy published a description of his work with 'dephlogisticated nitrous air'. Included within this work is a description of his personal use of the gas for pain relief, "I experienced an extensive inflammation of the gum, accompanied with great pain, which equally destroyed the power of repose and of consistent action. On the day when the inflammation was most troublesome, I breathed three large doses of nitrous oxide. The pain diminished after the first four or five respirations.....".[4]

Although nitrous oxide proved itself effective, it was partially replaced by ether (diethyl ether) and chloroform relatively quickly as these were available as volatile liquids which produced an inhalable vapour, and proved to be more potent anaesthetics. Early methods of delivering volatile anaesthetics using a soaked rag or sponge held over the patient's face inevitably often led to the surgeon, anaesthetist, and other operating room personnel receiving nearly the same dose of anaesthetic as the patient. Early this century reports from German researchers raised concerns over possible adverse effects of anaesthetic gases among health professionals[5,6] and led to some early attempts to divert waste gases and vapours away from those working in operating theatres. However, it was not until the 1960s and 1970s that this issue attracted much more attention when an epidemiological study

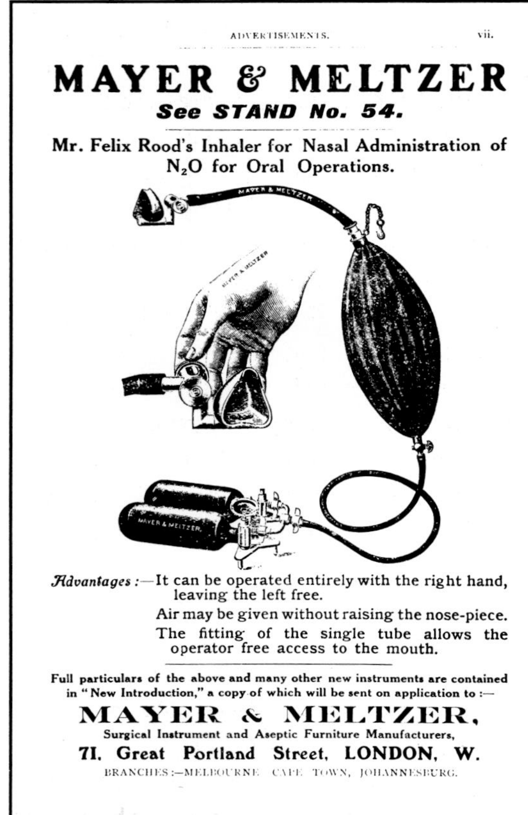

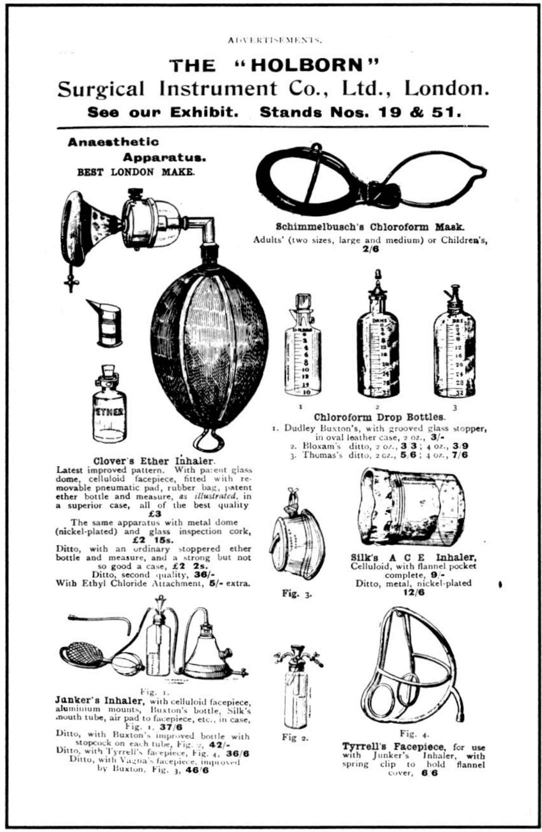

Anaesthetic equipment, circa 1910

of Soviet anaesthetists described adverse effects of headaches, fatigue and pruritus possibly resulting from poor working conditions.[7]

Although the discovery of anaesthetics seemed to provide a solution to the pain of childbirth, evidence increased as to the dangers involved in giving anaesthetics to mothers in labour. In 1929 the BMA's Anaesthetics in Midwifery Committee was appointed to consider the use of anaesthetics, analgesic and sedative drugs in childbirth, and to submit its findings, if urgent, to the Ministry of Health. It found that prolonged use of anaesthetic could cause delayed chloroform poisoning in the mother and that this was probably the real cause of many deaths ascribed to obstetric shock. The Committee's report concluded that "the indiscriminate use of chloroform or other anaesthetic would increase maternal mortality."[8]

Tragedies among x-ray pioneers

The discovery of x-rays was followed by a similar pattern of use to that of anaesthetics, with widespread application followed by a realisation of the dangers and consequent precautions taken, sadly too late for some. Röntgen discovered the x-ray or 'Röntgen ray' in 1895 and its diagnostic uses were realised remarkably swiftly. In the enthusiasm which followed, the rays were credited with many powers, some rather less credible than others. A New

York newspaper reported that, "at the college for physicians and surgeons, the Röntgen rays were used to reflect anatomic diagrams directly into the brains of the students, making a much more enduring impression than the ordinary methods of learning anatomical details."[9] The uses of radiation seemed endless, from treating ringworm to fitting shoes. Even up to the 1970s this latter practice persisted in some shoe shops. Staff using shoe-fitting fluoroscopes lacked training in radiation safety, and there were often no checks or controls on their use of the equipment.

At first, x-rays were believed to be harmless. However, within a year of the discovery, one side effect had become apparent; skin, hair and exposed parts of the body suffered if the rays reached them in any quantity. A painful kind of 'sunburn' appeared, the fingernails stopped growing and the eyelashes began to fall out. Interestingly, Sir Joseph Lister himself had suspected the danger. In 1896 he warned that, "the transmission of rays through the human body may not be altogether a matter of indifference to internal organs, but may by long continued action produce, according to the condition of the part concerned, injurious irritation or salutary stimulation."[10] But his words seem not to have been heeded.

In these early days of diagnostic radiology, x-ray tubes functioned erratically because of the varying gas content. Radiologists would commonly take several preliminary exposures of their hands to test the machine. Consequently many radiologists suffered ill effects and died prematurely. After some time the radiologist would notice that the skin on his hand was becoming cracked, red and inflamed. The acute symptoms would wear off but a roughened skin would persist. Eventually this would develop into cancer and a succession of amputations followed beginning with the fingertips and extending up the arms and ultimately death would result from the spread of the skin cancer to the internal organs.

International recommendations for x-ray and radiation protection were not issued until 1929, and even then only at the insistence of the British Committee at the International Congress of Radiology in Stockholm in 1928. The Society of Radiographers played an important part in regulating the use of radiation. Founded in 1920, the society emphasised the need for assistants installing and using x-ray equipment to be adequately trained, "in view of the terrible potentialities for evil which are universally acknowledged as belonging to the x-rays when handled in an unskilful manner."[11]

Public and occupational health

The effects of certain occupations on the health of their workforces have been observed over many years. Yet the idea that centralised action was necessary to control some of the dangers associated with workplace technology did not gain acceptance until the early 19th century, and even then there was considerable opposition to the aims of the reformers. The public health movement, which arose at this time, concerned itself not only with sanitary reform — clean water, effective sewage disposal and proper housing — but also with dangers encountered at work. Many of those concerned with public health issues, such as Lord Shaftesbury and Edwin Chadwick, fervently campaigned for improvements in factory conditions with considerable success. Despite Sir Robert Peel's factory legislation, the Health and Morals Apprentices Act (1802), which concerned hours of work, standards of cleanliness and education, injuries and deaths caused by factory machinery continued to be common. Some workers became physically deformed from working in cramped conditions or from long hours carrying out repetitive actions. In 1844 The Factories Act laid down regulations for fencing and protecting machinery, and three years later further legislation was introduced to regulate the hours and conditions of work for women and children.

Legislation required enforcement and following the 1833 Act to Regulate the Labour of Children and Young Persons in the Mines and Factories of the United Kingdom, four factory inspectors were appointed. Involvement of the medical profession in factory inspection soon followed. In 1834 Robert Baker, a medical practitioner, was appointed as sub-inspector of factories in Leeds, but the official post of Medical Inspector was not created until 1898. Dr Legge, the first to fill this post, was appointed by Sir Arthur Whitelegg, the Chief Inspector of Factories, who was himself a doctor.[12]

The provision of public health services exemplified by the appointment of Medical Officers of Health in local authorities throughout the UK, was well established by the middle of the 19th century. Certifying surgeons, who ascertained whether young persons entering factories were at least nine years old, were appointed under an 1844 Factory Act to investigate accidents at work. This latter duty was subsequently transferred to the Medical Inspectorate.

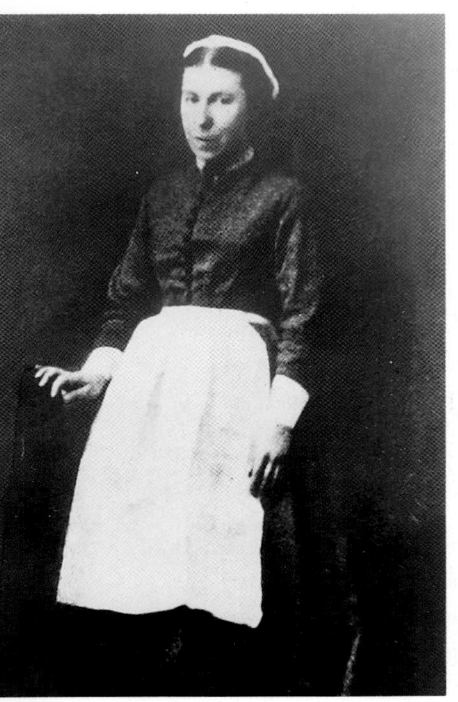
Philippa Flowerday, an early industrial nurse, appointed by Coleman's of Norwich in 1878

The appointment of the first Medical Inspector gave a lead to the establishment of a full time Medical Inspectorate for factories. These appointments are now embodied in the Employment Medical Advisory Service (EMAS) established in 1973, and subsumed within the Health and Safety Executive the following year. Employment Medical Advisors now have legal right of entry into all workplaces and have certain statutory responsibilities. The Health and Safety at Work etc Act (1974) provided a new legislative framework for health and safety in Britain, creating two new institutions — the Health and Safety Commission (HSC) and the Health and Safety Executive (HSE) — and integrated all inspection work under their control.

One of the first occupational health nurses appointed in the UK was at the Middlesborough Ironworks of Snowdon Hopkins & Co[13] in about 1858. Philippa Flowerday was appointed as one of the early industrial nurses to Colemans of Norwich in 1878. The appointment of medical officers or works' doctors in factories followed during the latter part of the 19th century and continues today. In both world wars the development of occupational health services was hastened by anxieties about the effect of ill health on production rates in ammunition factories.

Nowadays extensive legislation exists to protect the health of both employees and patients. The Health and Safety at Work etc Act (1974) and

legislation from the European Community set enforceable standards. Since the removal of Crown immunity from the NHS, the Health and Safety Executive may prosecute both the NHS Trust as a corporate body and individual managers where statutory standards are breached.

Under the Control of Substances Hazardous to Health (COSHH) Regulations (1988) employers are now required to assess the risk to health arising from exposure to hazardous substances. They must also ensure that exposure is adequately controlled and employees adequately informed about risks and safe systems of work[14] but these requirements have not always been diligently carried out. Thus today's challenges lie not in a lack of legislation, but in its implementation. Resources are needed to monitor its adherence and health care professionals and their employers must be convinced of the importance of these comprehensive regulations. For areas where legislation is not appropriate, guidelines can be drawn up, and these in turn mean that staff need educating about their use.

Hospital-acquired infection

In the past the dangers of working in health care, although not the subject of great public campaigns, were considerable. Throughout the 19th and early part of the 20th century, serious and even fatal infections acquired by doctors, nurses and other health staff in the course of medical practice were common. With the turn of the century, hospital-acquired infection, especially tuberculosis, continued to pose a major problem. At the Trudeau Sanatorium in New York between 1920 and 1953 as many as nine percent of the tuberculosis patients were themselves doctors or medical students[15]. Until the introduction of antibiotics, chest hospitals and sanatoria usually offered staff specially nourishing diets to strengthen their immunity.

With improvements in hygiene and the introduction of antibiotics, mortality rates from hospital-acquired infections were greatly reduced, but morbidity remained substantial. It is now estimated that 5%[16] of patients

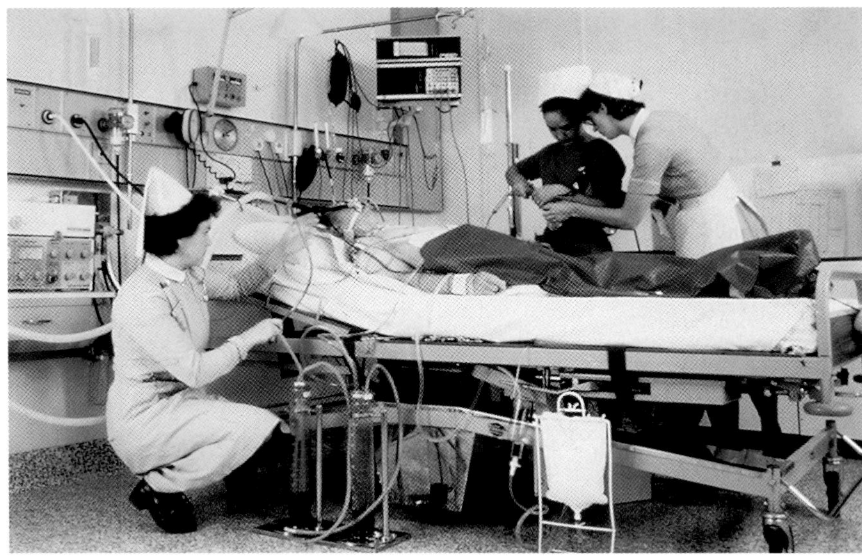

Hospital acquired infection remains a risk despite the introduction of modern medical practices

acquire an infection while in hospital — a figure which has not fallen over the past decade despite technological advances.

While the advent of antibiotics seemed to put an end to the great threat of infectious disease, the smooth line of progress proved once more to be illusory. New challenges have arisen in the changing patterns of illness among patients, antimicrobial resistance, and the inherent adaptability of many micro-organisms. The emergence of HIV and AIDS has brought new problems to the health care profession, tuberculosis is making a comeback, and viral hepatitis continues to be an important hazard. As health care advances to address these challenges, the education of staff in the occupational and environmental risks of health care is now more necessary than ever.

History shows that the introduction of new medical practices must be handled with care. It may transpire in the future that technologies and processes used today are less safe than we may think, and for this reason the research and review process must continue once an innovation is introduced into practice.

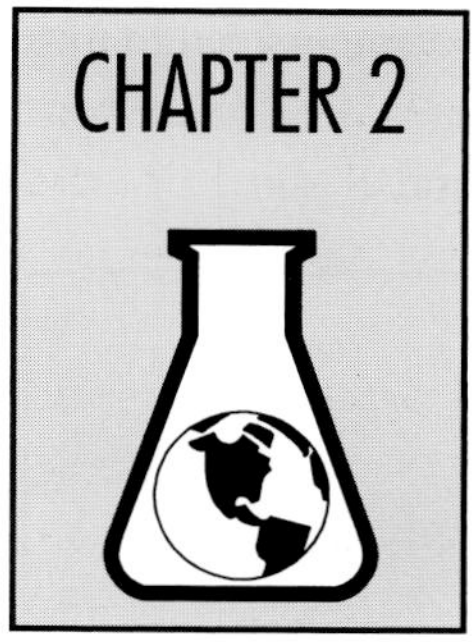

Environmental toxicology

This chapter aims to explain the functions and processes of environmental toxicology. It reaches beyond the scope of health care to serve as a general background to the following chapters.

Toxicology can be defined as the study and safety evaluation of chemicals and physical agents and the manner in which they gain entry into living organisms. It studies their effects from the molecular structure to the population level and the protective responses they induce. Environmental toxicology employs the same principles but addresses these mechanisms within the environment.

When a toxicologist investigates pharmaceutical drugs, the substance under investigation is already known, but within the environment, the hazard must first be detected before an assessment of the risk may be made. A hazard is the potential of a physical or chemical agent to do harm, and a risk is the probability that harm will be done under a given set of circumstances. The application of this process and the subsequent management of the identified risk may differ greatly however, because of the wide differences in what remedial action is considered feasible, generally acceptable and economic.[1]

According to the classic method,[2,3] the first step is to identify the hazard, and then to characterise it. This will require investigation of its nature and the dose and time response relation. A 'dose' is the quantity taken up at a given time, for instance, 50 micrograms of lead over one week. 'Exposure' is the total dose multiplied by the period of time (duration) over which man is in contact with the agent. The 'dose time response relation' is how a person responds to a particular dose over a given time. The effects of exposure may be delayed, as in the case of the 'slow virus' (prion) causing Creutzfeldt Jakob disease where the onset of dementia may be many years after infection. In such instances it can be difficult to trace the source of exposure due to the time lapse. Subsequently, the target population has to be identified and its exposure determined or predicted.

This process should permit reasonably confident assessment of the risk in terms of how many individuals will be affected (both absolute numbers or incidence) and what the harmful effects on them will be. By that stage the toxicologist may consider that his professional task has been completed, and he can leave to others such as politicians or administrators to decide on the acceptability of the risk and its management. This means balancing the personal, public and financial benefits of a new substance or procedure against individual, community, societal and environmental costs.

Steps in assessing risk

- Identify the hazard
- Identify the population at risk
- Characterise the hazard by investigating its nature and dose (time) response relation
- Determine or predict that population's exposure in terms of dose and duration
- Predict outcome

Although in theory all environmental toxicologists should subscribe to this model, it is not clear how reliable or accurate it is.

Hazard identification

To ensure a complete identification of a hazard this should include not only the known toxic hazard being investigated, the identity of the likely causal substance, and the relation between exposure and effect but also the characteristics of the population being studied.

Each of these factors may pose difficulties in assessing environmental toxicity as compared, say, to the conventional model of a dose of a drug. These difficulties arise because at the outset of investigations, there are so many unknown factors. The target population must be identified and characterised, as well as the substance they are exposed to. Evaluating the toxic effects in the population or in a more convenient laboratory model is a complex process.

Known toxic action

Hazards are usually characterised in laboratory models, because of the artifice of simplicity that is needed in the study of biological systems. This applies particularly to the investigation of toxicity due to exposure to air- or water-borne pollutants, or to contaminants in food. In the cases of air and water so many factors may be involved that outside the controlled

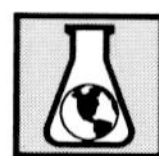

environment of the laboratory it is difficult to isolate those which are relevant.

Man is the target population with which we are concerned. However, in the usual route to identifying and characterising hazards, man's place is taken by laboratory animals. Findings can be hindered by physiological differences between species and the differences in toxic mechanisms and responses. For example, a resting adult human has a tidal respiratory volume of about 0.7l and a minute volume of, 6-8l when breathing at a rate of 10 to 12 breaths a minute. At rest a rat will breathe at a rate of about 120 to 150 inspirations a minute, with a tidal volume of about 1-1.5ml, and hence a minute volume of up to 200ml. This high rate will greatly affect exposure of laboratory animals to dusts and vapours — the sites and quantities deposited — and the penetration of water soluble toxicants down the respiratory tract, because a much higher proportion of the inhaled material may be deposited and absorbed from the upper respiratory tract by the rodent than in man.[4]

Laboratory animal experiments are essential in investigating such hazards, but interpretation of the results and their extrapolation to man are not straightforward. Lifespan can also confound findings. For instance, in chronic toxicity studies, where the aim is to discover the long term effects of a substance, rodents age far sooner than humans, since their lives are shorter. Towards the end of their lifespan, geriatric change results in a loss of sensitivity of these assessments. For this and other reasons, much of the literature on airborne toxic risks and standards is based on direct human experience, involving epidemiological and ecological surveys of residents or workers exposed while going about their daily lives.[5]

A related question is which toxic action is to be considered as the hazard. Atmospheric irritants may, for example, cause swelling of the eyes, watering of the eyes and of the nose, sneezing, nasal stuffiness, sore throat, cough and ultimately, perhaps, bronchitis and its secondary conditions. Which of these symptoms and conditions should be considered as the 'target' or 'indicator' action of relevance in identifying the hazard? In differing circumstances each will be important, but some are so trivial and occur so commonly that they may not necessarily be reliable indicators.

Examples of this type of difficulty are provided by the discussion on nitric oxide in a World Health Organisation (WHO) publication in 1987[6] and on ozone in a 1991 report from the Department of Health's Advisory Group on the Medical Aspects of Air Pollution.[7]

Exposure

In any attempt at an overall assessment of exposure to a polluted environment, it is necessary to consider uptake by respiration (reasonably straightforward), by absorption through the skin, by oral ingestion — either coughed up and swallowed deposits from the respiratory tree, or (and much less certain) the amounts deposited from the air on food (plants) or ingested by animals from whom food is prepared. The latter routes may appear

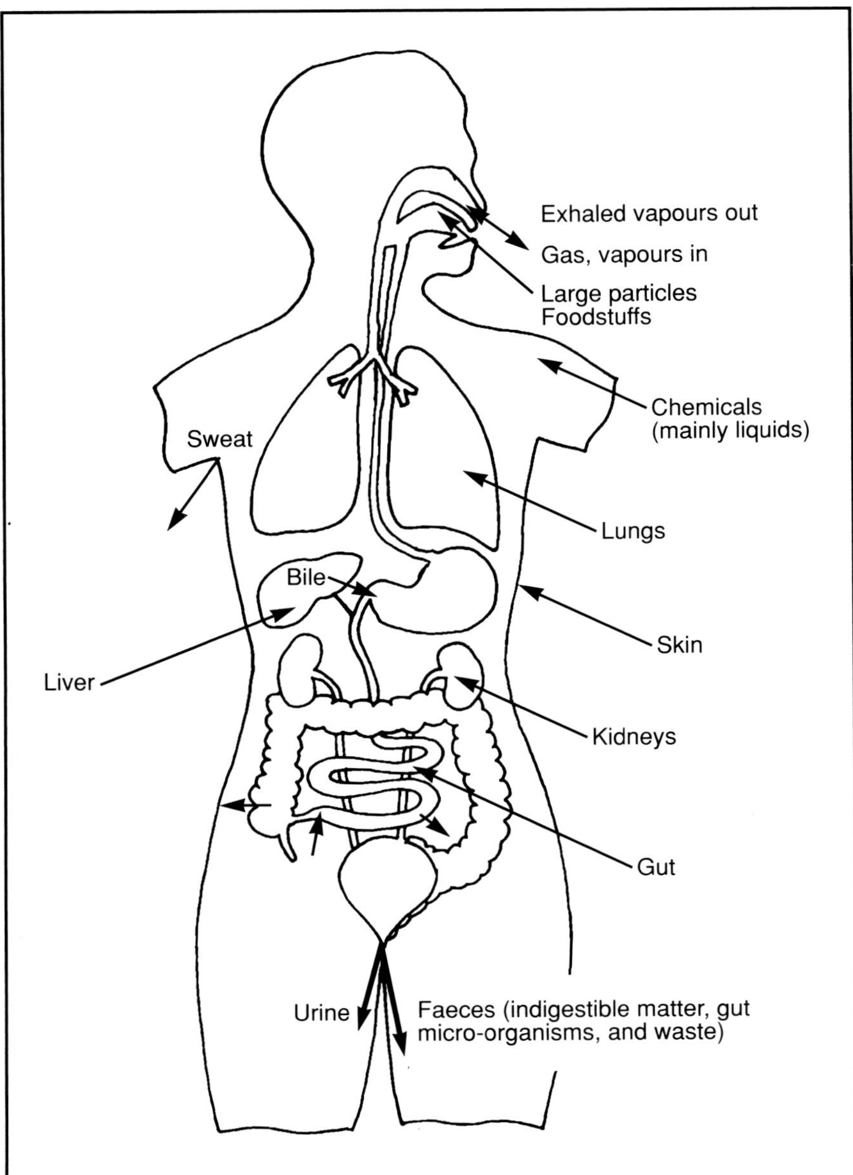

Figure 2.1: Toxic substances enter the body by respiration, absorption through the skin, by ingestion or by absorption through the gut. Once absorbed, they are metabolised or 'broken down' and eventually excreted through exhaled vapours, sweat, urine and faeces.

insignificant but experience of radioactive fallout has shown that they cannot be ignored.

Some of the potential uncertainties in determining exposure at the site of action have been mentioned above. There is also the difficulty of knowing what degree exposure to a toxicant is relevant. Thus not only might the average, peak, and total duration of exposure (and time envelope if intermittent) be relevant data, but so too is the analytical method and model used to assess the several pollutants commonly found in air. For example, industrial contamination may give rise to nitrous oxide, ozone and sulphur dioxide, and acidified water droplets, both free and absorbed onto soot particles. All are likely to contribute to the potential of city air to cause harm, but do they act individually or in combination? And if the latter, is the outcome additive or synergistic?[8,9]

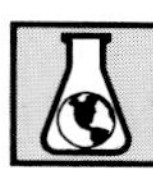

Analyses of urban air, and no less of indoor air, are marked by the multiplicity of potential toxicants found, ranging from simple inorganic compounds, such as the classical nitrates and ozone, to more or less complex organic chemicals, including formaldehyde, complex nitriles and polycyclic aromatic hydrocarbons.[10,11] Furthermore, the proximity of combustion sources and motor vehicles, means that 1,3 butadiene, benzene and other aromatics may also be significant pollutants.[12,13] Thus, critical identification, even of airborne hazards, requires careful consideration of what substances might be present, in what concentration, and under what circumstances, in order to identify the important components in any given circumstance.

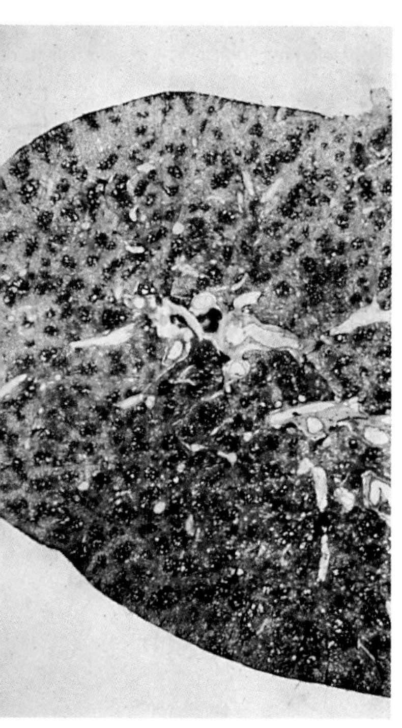

The industrial disease pneumoconisosis can be caused by small particles becoming trapped in the lungs. Here, coal dust has caused the disease shown in this section of lung tissue

Particles small enough to reach the lungs (respirable particles) also pose a danger. Silica is such a particle and can cause a kind of pneumoconiosis; an industrial disease. These particles become trapped and irritate the lung causing damage eg the development of fibrous tissue.

Waterborne pollutants may at first appear simpler to deal with, but in reality they form at least as complex a mixture, and they too vary with time, often cyclically over the years. More than 1,000 chemicals have been identified in water at a low to very low level, some due to industrial pollution, many of natural origin, and others added during purification and distribution. They may be produced by the common disinfection process of chlorination, ozonolysis or ultra violet irradiation, as these act on natural and industrial pollutants.[14] The same general cautions apply, therefore, to any simplistic attempt to assess a particular hazard of water pollution.

Assessment of exposure is therefore complex. Exposure may occur via several routes to a number of different agents simultaneously, and they may additionally ameliorate or potentiate each others effects. Some of the complexities of predicting environmental pollution caused by industrial chemicals and of measuring what is present in air and water are discussed in an European Chemical Industry Ecology and Toxicology Centre (ECETOC) report published in 1988[15].

Mixed exposures

Exposure in practice is commonly to a mixture of substances and the consequence may represent simple summation of the action of each component, or, sometimes, the components may interact causing a different and usually enhanced effect. If someone were to encounter a mixture of simple irritants, such as formaldehyde and acid vapours, the inflammation caused in the skin, eyes or upper respiratory tract would usually be additive. However, the inhalation of a combination of sulphur dioxide and airborne particles, as in smog, will lead to increased irritation, probably because the acid gas is absorbed onto the particles so that a larger amount is carried further down the airways. Damage to the integrity of physical barriers in the body can also lead to a great increase in local and even systemic toxic actions, as in exposure of moist skin (for example, skin enclosed in gloves or soaked in water) to a toxicant, or if the skin has been damaged by an organic solvent.

Evidence is accumulating that certain pollutant gases, such as sulphur dioxide and ozone, impair an individual's respiratory defence mechanisms and so increase the incidence and perhaps the severity of bacterial and viral infections of the airways. The gases may also cause an increased incidence of sensitisation to aerial allergens, and comparable processes may operate in the skin. Physical agents may have a role, too, since natural ultra violet irradiation such as sunbathing can depress immunity in the skin perhaps exciting or exacerbating allergic dermatitis.

Toxicological experience covers many examples of systemic interactions occurring from various combinations of drugs and industrial chemicals, including, for example, pharmacological classics, such as aspirin, as well as enzyme inducers or inhibitors and warfarin and oral contraceptives. Few environmental pollutants are so active that such synergism or inhibition is likely after limited exposure, but longer-lived agents, such as dioxins and organochlorine pesticides have occasionally been suggested as the cause of unexpected changes in sensitivity. Unrealised cholinesterase inhibition by organophosphorous pesticides has also been known to cause over-reaction in patients subsequently treated therapeutically with a similar agent.[16,17]

The best general approach is always to consider the possibility of interactions when evaluating the potential harmfulness of a mixed exposure by taking account of the toxic load and properties of the individual components.

Risk assessment

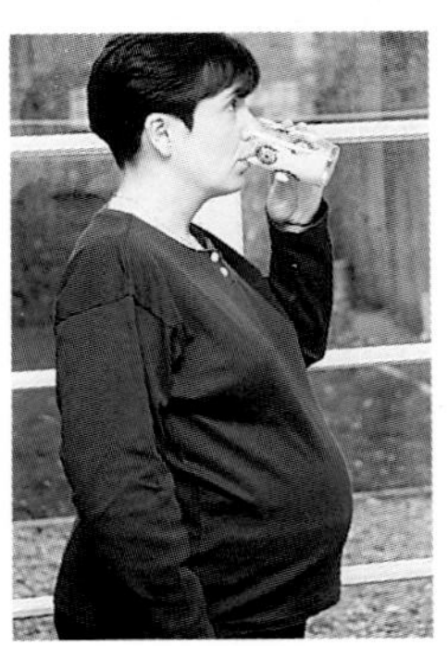

Environmental toxins may be particularly hazardous to the foetus

Risk assessment comprises auditing the exposure of the population affected as well as consideration of the exposure-response relationships in order to determine the incidence, nature and severity of the toxic action.

Exposure to an environmental toxin may affect anyone, so in practice it is necessary to consider the implications of a range of susceptibility (that may include the sex and age of the subject, the amount of exercise taken, and whether a woman is pregnant). Determining the risk to a foetus is particularly problematic. Hazards which may normally pose little or no threat to the population may cause foetal damage. For example, exposure of pregnant women to substances such as lead and mercury have been linked with birth defects.[18] Other factors affecting susceptibility, are the effects of genetic susceptibility, the general state of health, any pre-existing disease, prior or co-exposure to other toxic agents (including drugs, alcohol, chemicals at work, etc) and immune status including any true immunological hypersensitivity.[19]

Each of these factors separately or in various combinations may determine whether there is an effect at all, or its severity. The basis for deciding is a knowledge of the real population at risk rather than of an idealised and simplified version.[20,21] These data are not always available in detail, particularly because such a comprehensive assessment involves responses both from adults, and in respect of contemporary and

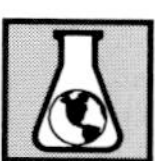

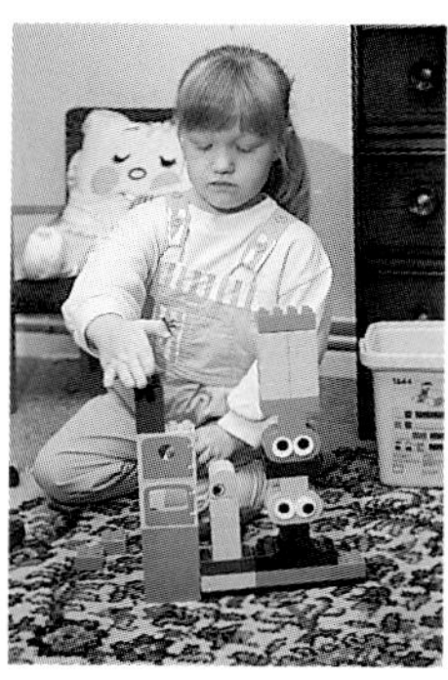

High levels of industrial pollution may affect children's growth

developmental concerns, for the young. To take atmospheric pollution as an example, recent interest has focused upon the idea that when children live in areas where the air contains much industrial pollution they not only suffer from the acute effects, but may show a higher than average incidence of asthma along with recurrent attacks of bronchitis and retardation in growth.[22] This could have important implications for affected children and the wider community by interrupting their schooling, thus lowering their educational attainments, which in turn could reduce the population's range of skills.

These effects may be related to total exposure, as in acute irritation of the upper airways, or their occurrence may appear stochastic in nature, as in the development of asthma and other forms of the hypersensitivity, where small numbers of individuals develop a disorder with little evidence of a conventional dose-response relationship.

Exposure standards in environmental toxicity

The complexities of evaluating the population at risk and the full range of exposures mean that it is difficult to predict accurately the effects in the general population. When setting a standard for control of a population exposure, it is important to base it as far as possible on evidence from the target species — man — by including epidemiological findings. It is also advisable to use a safety margin that allows for the distribution of susceptibilities and sensitive individuals in the population at risk. The principles and practical difficulties of this process are well illustrated by the recent account of the effects of ozone pollution from the Department of Health's advisory group[23] and the caution evident in the WHO's 1987 guidelines on air quality for Europe.[24]

The aim of setting standards is to ensure that exposure is so limited as to prevent any unacceptable harm to the population at risk. For instance, in setting the limits for pesticides, the level is set where there is 'no observable effect' in the most sensitive test species. These studies have to cover possible production of cancers of various types, birth and inheritance defects as well as effects on the nervous and reproductive systems. As already discussed, the problems are centred on exposure to a particular substance, how to measure this, and what actions it has in which people. Furthermore, controlling general exposure of the population to the environment is dependent on two factors. One is geography — for instance, the effect of mountains in channelling air, or use of surface or ground waters for drinking. The other is the effect that environmental decisions will have on industry and economic activity, a major source of pollutants. So setting standards requires careful and often difficult decisions that may influence the siting of a population and its work places. This will provoke powerful political and economic arguments as well as widespread anxieties about the community's health that are customarily the province of doctors and medical toxicologists.[25-27]

Discussion

The setting of 'standards' in science or medicine implies that an absolute level of a given substance or activity can be maintained. This suggests that complete control is possible at all times and under all circumstances. Such an outcome is difficult if not impossible to achieve in the case of environmental pollution. This is especially so for such a mobile and changeable medium as air, with seasonal climatic variations, air movement over long distances and temperature inversions in the atmosphere. Other factors are differences in concentration of pollutants indoors and outside, and variations in the age and activity of people which affects the proportion of time spent inside and outdoors — for example, the contrast between children playing in the open, and adults in a sedentary office occupation.

For these and other reasons, and to indicate their nature as best estimates for many substances, it is common to set 'Environmental Quality Objectives' or 'Guidance Values' to set exposures that should not be exceeded.

Lists of values for air and water pollutants have been published by several international and national agencies[28] and the EC.[29,30] These have attempted to reflect experimental and human data, mixed and fluctuating patterns of exposure, and the range of individuals in the population who might be affected. Not surprisingly, they differ in scope and in detail, because the values proposed often represent compromises between certainty and generous extrapolation.

Despite the limitations in our understanding of environmental toxicology, arising from its complexity and the short time during which it has been formally studied, the main routes of investigation and the principal goals are reasonably well established. This is true whether concerns encompass a continent or a country, or affect a conurbation, a particular industry or just a local plant. In common with other forms of toxicology, and despite the complexity of the source nature and distribution of environmental pollutants, we must consider the nature of the population at risk, evaluate the extent and duration of exposure (at rest, at work and at play), and then assess the likely adverse effects by reference to epidemiological findings and human and animal experimental results.

As the following chapters illustrate, there are many potential hazards in the health care sector facing workers, patients and the environment. To safeguard occupational and environmental health, comprehensive health and safety policies are required, many of which are already in place. These rely on accurate risk assessments, which, in turn, rely upon reliable toxicological information. Unless this information is gathered and then made available, hazards will remain unidentified. As health care becomes ever more complex and diverse, this important research should continue to be awarded a high priority.

CHAPTER 3

Chemicals used in the health care industry

Large amounts of chemical substances are used by modern industrialised countries and their use is increasing in developing countries. Soaps, detergents, perfumes, dyes, deodorants, cleaners, disinfectants, surfactants, propellants, therapeutic agents, and a host of other applications require chemicals for their production. The number of synthetic organic chemicals used and disposed of by society is increasing at a rate of about 1000 new chemicals a year.

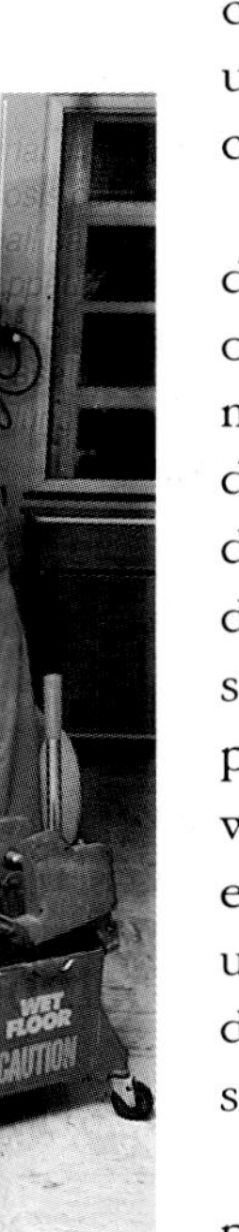

Many chemicals, including bleaches, detergents and polishes are used in hospitals

In the health care sector the proliferation of chemicals has mirrored developments in society. Examples include, the cleansing and disinfection of endoscopes and surgical equipment, preoperative skin preparation, medicines and cement for joint replacements. Many are necessary for the direct care of patients, but chemicals are also used in other ways. Not only do hospital laboratories require large amounts of preservatives, fixatives, dyes, and cleaning and disinfectant agents but hospitals also provide 'hotel' services that need cleansers, detergents, bleaches, washing powders, polishes, and other products. Many hospitals contain 'industrial' zones in which chemicals are used. Examples are boilerhouses, metal fabrication, electronic equipment, waste disposal, and other support services, where the use of chemicals may differ from that in clinical areas. General medical and dental practices, too, need chemicals for the effective provision of their services.

Medical care is supported by a large industry supplying all the necessary products and processes, and some of the world's largest companies manufacture medicines, and medical equipment and appliances, for which a host of chemicals are required. Even the manufacture of something as simple and as frequently used as a sticky plaster requires numerous chemicals to make the absorbent material, plastic, adhesive, and sealed package which together comprise the finished, sterilised product.

Controlling exposure

Classically, harmful exposure may arise in several ways: by inhalation of fumes or vapours (important for gases and volatile liquids), absorption through the skin (particularly of fat soluble substances), or ingestion and absorption from the gut. Exposure of workers to many harmful chemicals is controlled in the UK by legislation such as the Health and Safety at Work etc Act (1974) and the Control of Substances Hazardous to Health Regulations (COSHH 1988), and statutory exposure limits published yearly.[1] Assessment of exposure has historically been made by measuring airborne levels of harmful substances, and most of the exposure criteria are framed in this way. The measurement of the dose of a chemical actually absorbed (biological monitoring) or its effect on the body (biological effect monitoring) are relatively new techniques and as yet are hard to interpret. In the UK exposure limits may be defined as mean exposure during an eight hour shift (an eight hour time-weighted average), or if short but relatively high levels of exposure are thought to be important in causing adverse effects, over a 10 minute exposure period (10 minute short term exposure limit). Two types of exposure limit may be set. One, the occupational exposure standard (OES), is the more common and it defines a level of airborne exposure which should not be exceeded, or if exceeded the reasons should be identified and remedied as soon as reasonably practicable. The other is a maximum exposure limit (MEL), which is more usual where a safe level of exposure cannot be clearly defined (as with most carcinogens) and which requires exposure to be reduced as far as reasonably practicable, and to be kept at all times below the level set.

The growth in health care technology and its accompanying use of chemicals has increased the potential risk of damage to health service employees and to the environment outside the workplace. Any harmful consequences will depend on the dose and pattern of employees' exposure, and the amount and nature of any releases to the environment. It is a matter for concern that exposure limits are based upon an eight hour period while most junior doctors continue to work for much longer periods within the hospital environment. Prolonged exposure to such chemicals from extended working times should be considered in setting limits and allocating workload. Greater public awareness of such issues has prompted consideration of how these chemicals affect human health and the environment and led to a wealth of legislation to protect employees and the environment.

Chemicals used in health care

Given that nearly all health care in the UK is provided by the NHS, it might be imagined that safety data on its use of chemicals would be readily available. This is not so. Not only is the NHS geographically fragmented and made up of numerous separate hospitals and clinics, but also many professionals work as independent contractors for the NHS providing

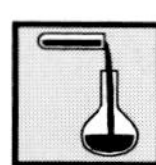

general medical and dental services. Some District Health Authorities have merged and still more are in the process of doing so. Information on the type and total amount of chemicals purchased by the health service is difficult to obtain.

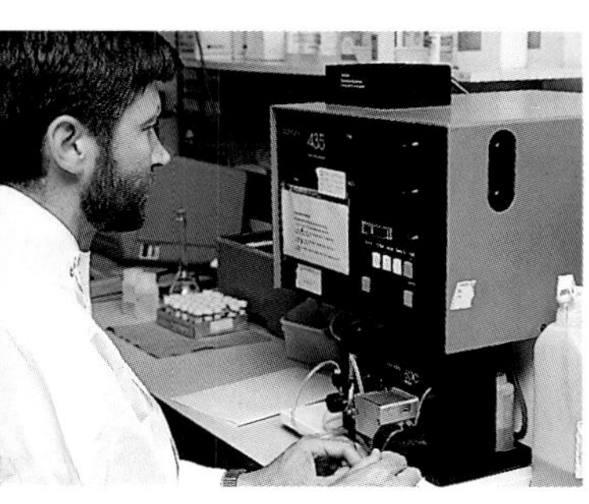

Health care workers and laboratory staff may be exposed routinely to a range of chemicals

Certain chemicals used within health care have repeatedly prompted concern. These are usually chemicals associated with health care rather than 'hotel' functions. However, because most chemicals used in the 'hotel' functions are similar to those used in the home, (except that they may be more concentrated), this may mean that staff handle them too complacently. Little is known about any possible effects from their use in health care, either in terms of exposure in the workplace or in the environment. A number of these products do however, contain recognised irritants and sensitisers, and consequently skin problems among cleaners, food preparation staff, maintenance workers, and other domestic or hotel service staff are thought to be not uncommon.

Examples of chemicals that are recognised to cause such health problems include: hypochlorite bleaches and disinfectants; strongly alkaline cleaners; formaldehyde cleaners; epoxy resins used in glues and repair pastes; perfumes in soaps, detergents, shampoos, and air fresheners; enzymes in soap powders; lanolin in soaps and shampoos; and even constituents of

Potential problem substances used in NHS

- Glutaraldehyde and formaldehyde used as disinfectants and fixatives in laboratories and clinical areas, and in developing and fixing films in radiology departments
- Ethylene oxide used for sterilisation of surgical equipment
- Methyl methacrylate used in orthopaedic surgery, dentistry and chiropody
- Methanol, xylene, and propan-2-ol used as solvents and fixatives in pathology
- Mercury spillages from clinical equipment
- Solvents and inks used in printing
- Perchloroethylene used in workshops, laundries, and in printing
- Anaesthetic and analgesic gases
- Resin systems used in pathology for fixing specimens
- Several other chemicals including 1,1,1 trichloroethane, paraffin wax, dichloromethane, ozone (arising from ultraviolet therapy and photocopiers), carbon monoxide, solvent vapour from paints, dust from plaster of Paris and lightweight fibre casts, asbestos and wood dusts, and welding fumes.[2]

'protective' rubber gloves.[3] The overall burden of skin problems is not clearly established as this section of health care has been studied relatively infrequently, and many employees may be loath to report what they perceive as transient and mild problems with familiar products.

Occupational exposure to some chemicals, particularly those associated specifically with health care, has been studied in more detail. Even for these, however, little information is available about their possible environmental effects. The University of Birmingham's Institute of Occupational Health has provided an occupational health service for the West Midlands Regional Health Authority, including advice and help with occupational hygiene problems arising from the use of chemicals in the NHS. Recent inquiries to this service have identified several potential problem substances (see boxed text on page 25).

Although not comprehensive, this list emphasises the breadth of daily activities in health care and hence the wide range of chemicals used — many in substantial amounts — that are potentially damaging both to employees' health and to the environment. Many of these chemicals are used in industry and are not exclusive to the NHS. Experience from industrial usage may be a valuable source of knowledge. Because of the wide range of chemicals used and lack of information available this section cannot provide a comprehensive review of all chemicals used in health care, or in the production of its technological equipment. Instead, this section focuses on four chemicals that are a common cause of concern. These are formaldehyde, glutaraldehyde, ethylene oxide and methyl methacrylate. The levels of exposure quoted use the same units as reported in the source documents.

Formaldehyde

Several chemicals used in health care are utilised elsewhere in industry. Formaldehyde, for example, is a constituent of urea/formaldehyde resin adhesives and of permanent-press fabrics. It is utilised, too, in the manufacture of textiles, rubber, photographic film, leather, and cosmetics. Urea/formaldehyde resin systems are essential in various industrial processes, such as binding the moulds used for casting metal in foundries. So not surprisingly, formaldehyde production worldwide runs to many thousands of metric tons. Table 3.1 shows an estimate of production in 1981 and this has probably increased since then.[4] Because formaldehyde is such a common chemical in industry its use in health care probably represents only a small proportion of total use. The present exposure limit in the UK is 2.0ppm (as a 10 minute short term maximum exposure limit (MEL) — this limit should not be exceeded).

Exposure to formaldehyde has been associated with several adverse effects. Skin or mucous membranes may become inflamed if the concentration is sufficiently strong, with concentrations as low as 0.1-0.3ppm being associated with symptoms. Most people however, will not react until concentrations reach 2-3ppm.[5] Concentrations of 10ppm can

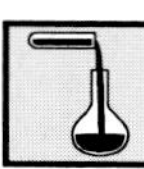

Table 3.1
Estimated worldwide formaldehyde production 1981

Country	*Production (thousands of metric tons)*
Europe: EEC	
Belgium	31
Denmark	70
France	477
West Germany	2,292
Greece	72
Italy	900
Netherlands	311
Portugal	90
Spain	385
United Kingdom	496
Europe: non EEC	864
North America	
Canada	280
Mexico	90
USA	2,595
Japan	1,039
Other	997

Source: Martin PA, Cross HJ, Harrington JM. Formaldehyde : a report. Birmingham Institute of Occupational Health, 1986.

usually be tolerated for only a few minutes, and at 10-20ppm it may be difficult to breathe because of the acutely irritant effects of the chemical on the upper airways. Some studies suggest that some of the symptoms which characterise the 'sick building syndrome' may be caused by formaldehyde.[6,7]

It is present at very low concentrations as an environmental contaminant in many modern buildings because of 'off-gassing' from laminates, furniture, and insulation materials. (Off-gassing is the slow evaporation of residual chemicals from the structures and furnishings, etc.)

A study of symptoms among workers in two types of day care centres in Denmark found drowsiness, headache, upper respiratory tract irritation, eye irritation, and menstrual irregularities to be significantly more common in those working in mobile units where median concentrations of formaldehyde were higher than elsewhere.[8] Another study, specifically comparing histology technicians exposed to various chemicals, including formaldehyde, with a group of secretaries and clerks, reported significant

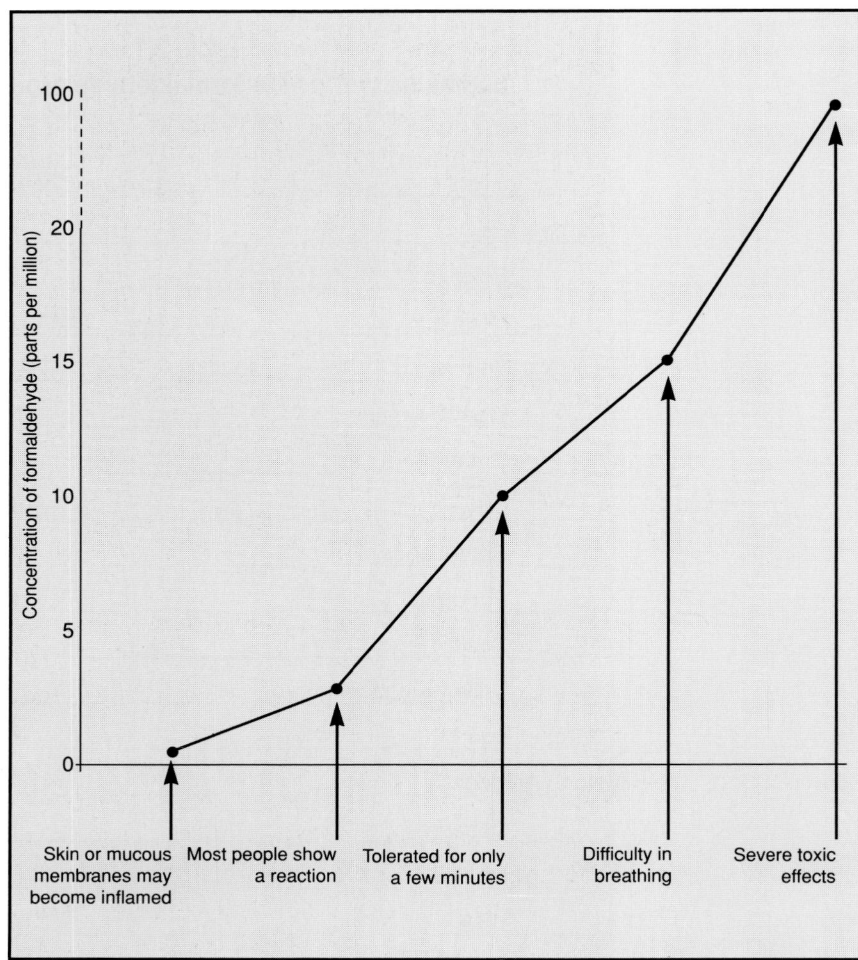

Figure 3.1: Adverse effects associated with exposure to increasing concentrations of formaldehyde in air

increases in certain symptoms among the technicians. These included lack of concentration, loss of memory, disturbed sleep, impaired balance, variations in mood, alterations of appetite, indigestion, nausea, headache, and fatigue.[9] A dose-response relationship was also found, the subjects' symptoms increasing with their daily duration of exposure to formaldehyde. Several other studies, however, have failed to confirm this hypothesis, the authors finding no relation between exposure to formaldehyde and some of the symptoms associated with sick building syndrome.[10,11]

Sensitisation and respiratory effects

Some researchers have found an association between formaldehyde exposure and respiratory disease. Kilburn et al[12] reported a significant increase in the frequency of chest tightness, cough, and 'burning' chest pain in histology technicians exposed to formaldehyde at concentrations of 0.2-1.9ppm when compared with a group of secretaries and clerks. The technicians were also exposed to other chemicals such as xylene and toluene.

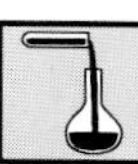

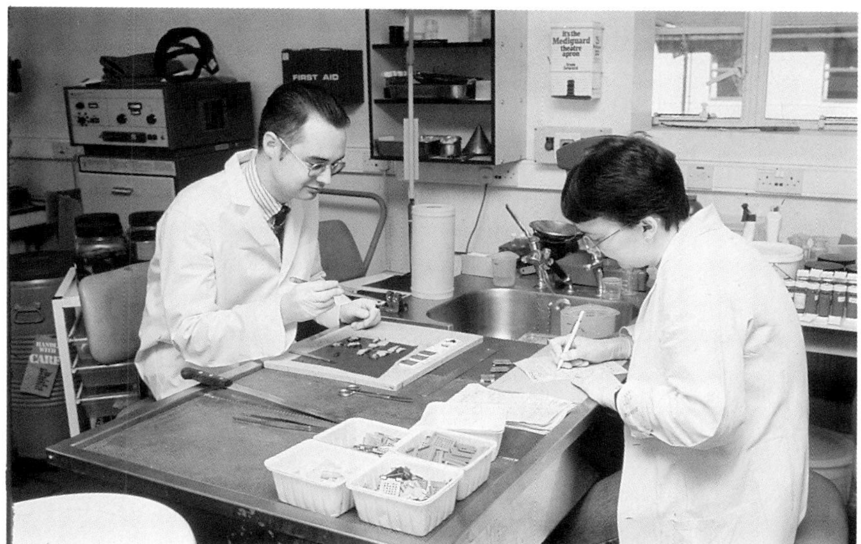

Histopathology technicians may be exposed to formaldehyde during specimen preparation

Formaldehyde has been identified as a cause of occupational asthma in health care workers, the first such description relating to a 41 year-old nursing sister in a dialysis unit.[13] Investigation of the other staff on the same unit identified another nurse with occupational asthma caused by exposure to formaldehyde (proved by specific airway challenge).[14] The unit had 28 staff, and 6 others complained of at least one episode of respiratory symptoms, suggestive of asthma or bronchitis, since starting work in the dialysis unit, an overall prevalence of 29%. These studies did not report any measurements of exposure to formaldehyde, although a later report on 15 subjects with suspected formaldehyde-induced asthma did try to determine the levels of exposure which could precipitate an asthmatic reaction.[15] Symptoms and changes in lung function were precipitated at a mean exposure of 3.2ppm for 30 minutes, but they could occur in the most sensitised subjects after exposure to <0.3ppm for 30 minutes.

Two studies of exposure to formaldehyde in asthmatic subjects who had not previously been sensitised to formaldehyde have been reported. One found no changes in lung function among a group of 15 asthmatic subjects following exposures of 0.7ppm and 0.10ppm for approximately 90 minutes.[16] In the second, 15 asthma sufferers who had not been sensitised to formaldehyde were exposed to concentrations of formaldehyde of 2ppm for approximately 40 minutes.[17] No significant changes in symptoms or lung function were identified in the group following exposure, although a small increase in airway reactivity to methacholine was detected. (The relevance of this finding remains unclear although it may be important in the process of sensitisation.) These studies emphasise the importance of prior sensitisation in the expression of hypersensitivity to formaldehyde.

Formaldehyde can cause both an irritant and a hypersensitivity dermatitis when in direct contact with skin in sufficient concentrations.[18] Allergic dermatitis has been reported among nurses handling 100g/l solutions of formaldehyde, as well as among staff in a dialysis unit using 20g/l solutions to sterilise open tanks.[19]

Carcinogenicity

Uncertainty exists over whether formaldehyde is carcinogenic in humans. It has mutagenic effects on micro-organisms and insects, an action thought to be an important step in carcinogenesis. It is almost certainly carcinogenic in some animals, exposures of 6-15ppm being associated with nasal tumours in rats and mice.[20-23] In humans, however, the evidence is inconclusive. A study of chromosome aberrations and sister chromatid exchange in the lymphocytes of staff in pathology departments showed no differences in these markers of genetic damage between exposed and unexposed individuals.[24] Studies of pathologists and medical laboratory technicians in Britain have suggested that this group may have an above average incidence of deaths from lymphatic and haemopoietic neoplasms, and brain cancers. There was no rise above the expected occurrence of cancers of the lung, nose, or nasal sinuses as animal evidence had suggested might be the case.[25-27]

The International Agency for Research on Cancer (IARC) has concluded that the body of data suggests sufficient evidence to implicate formaldehyde as a carcinogen in animals but that there was limited evidence for its carcinogenicity in humans; the agency classified the chemical as a class 2A carcinogen.[28] Given that some doubt remains about the carcinogenicity of formaldehyde, it is hard to make any relevant estimate of the risk of any given level of exposure.

International Agency for Research on Cancer
Evaluations of carcinogenic risk to humans

Class	
1	Agent is carcinogenic to humans
2A	Agent is probably carcinogenic to humans
2B	Agent is possibly carcinogenic to humans
3	Not classified as to carcinogenicity in humans
4	Agent is probably not carcinogenic in humans[29]

Exposure

Various levels of exposure to formaldehyde have been reported for health care workers performing certain tasks. The chemical is probably most used as a preservative and disinfectant in pathology and anatomy departments and one paper has described environmental levels of formaldehyde in 10 histopathology laboratories in California.[30] Air samples were collected using

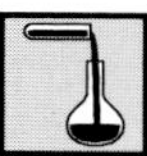

static samplers at different positions in 10 of the 25 laboratories studied over a period of one to four hours. Formaldehyde concentrations in tissue specimen preparation and sampling areas ranged from 0.2-1.9ppm. The paper contrasted this exposure with that of subjects in areas of clerical and office work, where air sampling showed no detectable concentrations of formaldehyde. A similar study of formaldehyde concentration in eight anatomy teaching laboratories in a medical school reported readings of 0.3-2.6ppm.[31] A study of personal exposures of pathologists and technicians in an autopsy room, using a personal sampler to estimate concentrations of formaldehyde in the breathing zone of subjects, found measurements of 0.61-1.32ppm (eight hour time-weighted average), with peak concentrations exceeding 3.0ppm on several occasions.[32] Another study of a hospital morgue in Canyon City, Colorado, found an average personal exposure of 4.8ppm (eight hour time-weighted average estimated using personal samplers).[33]

Formaldehyde solution is used to clean and disinfect the internal hoses of haemodialysis machines, and for disinfection of equipment in peritoneal dialysis. Ambient samples from five dialysis clinics in the USA showed:

- The highest mean formaldehyde concentration of 0.27ppm (range 0.06-0.92ppm) in the area of a drain used during cleaning of equipment
- A mean exposure concentration of 0.13ppm (range 0.02-0.37ppm) in the area of the nurses' station
- A mean exposure concentration of 0.11ppm (range 0.02-0.65ppm) next to the dialysis machine
- A surprisingly high figure of 0.9ppm in a utility room used for storage.[34]

Other studies have reported similar exposures, one reporting concentrations of up to 0.9ppm in dialysis units in hospitals in San Francisco,

Table 3.2
Reported exposures to formaldehyde

Place/process	*Mean exposure (ppm)*	*Reference**
Mortuary	4.80	Daniels
Pathology		
Specimen prepartion	0.2-1.9	Kilburn
Cadaver dissection	0.61-1.32 (peak >3.0)	Coldiron
Anatomy laboratory	0.3-2.6	Skisak
Haemodialysis	0.02-0.92	Smith

*For full details see chapter reference list.

Table 3.3
Typical formaldehyde exposures for several processes/activities

Department	Process	Sample type	Sampling period (mins)	Concentration (ppm)	(mg/m^3)
Pathology	making up 10% solution	personal	2	2.0	(2.5)
		static	2	2.0	(2.5)
		personal	32	0.46	(0.58)
		static	32	1.2	(1.5)
	decanting into specimen pots	personal	20	0.17	(0.21)
		static	20	0.36	(0.45)
	specimen trimming (with extraction)	personal	26	0.24	(0.3)
		personal	25	0.26	(0.33)
		personal	16	0.006	(0.007)
		personal	16	0.009	(0.011)
		personal	37	2.2	(2.7)
		static	37	2.59	(3.24)
		static	37	2.7	(3.37)
	photographing specimen	personal	20	1.25	(1.56)
		static	20	6.87	(8.59)
	throw out	personal	21	1.82	(2.28)
		personal	20	1.92	(2.4)
		personal	22	4.34	(5.45)
		static	30	5.33	(6.66)
		personal	31	not detected	
		personal	21	1.5	(1.9)
		static	21	10.5	(13.1)
Endoscopy		personal	25	0.23	(0.29)
		static	23	0.17	(0.21)
		static	50	0.03	(0.04)
		static	15	0.14	(0.17)
Radiology	processing	static	various	not detected	

Source: Exposures measured by Occupational Health Unit, West Midlands Regional Health Authority, Institute of Occupational Health, University of Birmingham.

and another concentration, of 0.04-0.50ppm at a peritoneal dialysis unit in Cincinnati.[35,36] A summary of some reported levels of exposure to formaldehyde is shown in table 3.2.

It is hard to find any reports on concentrations of formaldehyde in health units in the United Kingdom. Data collected by the Occupational Health Unit of West Midlands Regional Health Authority showed that typical levels of exposure to formaldehyde during various processes are below exposure limits (table 3.3).[37] Sometimes, this limit may be exceeded during processes

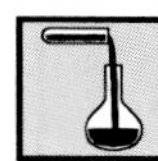

such as trimming specimens, particularly large postmortem specimens, photographing large postmortem specimens under hot lights, preparing dilute solutions of formaldehyde and disposing of used formalin.

There are no reports of concentrations of possible external environmental contamination arising from formaldehyde use in the health service. It has to be disposed of through drainage and ventilation systems, but because formaldehyde occurs naturally, it would be difficult to estimate the contribution of health service waste to its presence in the environment. Disposal of other health service waste may also add to this problem. For example, the incineration of plastic syringes may produce formaldehyde.

Glutaraldehyde

Glutaraldehyde may be used outside health care as a tanning agent for leather and as a preservative in cosmetics. It came into widespread use in health care later than formaldehyde and it is less commonly used in industry than formaldehyde. Thus less information is available about its possible adverse effects, even so, some have been identified. One paper described effects occurring in endoscopy unit staff cleaning instruments in 2% glutaraldehyde.[38] Reported effects in these staff included watering of the eyes, rhinitis, breathlessness, and dermatitis. Another paper has also described local irritant and non specific symptoms such as nasal catarrh and obstruction, smarting of the throat, headache, and nausea occurring significantly more frequently among health care workers regularly exposed to glutaraldehyde than among a group who were less exposed.[39] Again, these symptoms occurred despite exposure below current UK limits. The current UK exposure limit is 0.2ppm (10 minute short term exposure limit). Glutaraldehyde has often been reported to cause dermatitis, both among workers in endoscopy units exposed to a 2% solution and in radiology staff exposed to glutaraldehyde used in processing films;[40-42] irritant and allergic (or hypersensitivity) mechanisms are probably involved.

Respiratory effects

Adverse effects to the respiratory tract have been reported after exposure to glutaraldehyde. It is soluble in water and dissolves rapidly in respiratory mucus, so tending to cause irritant symptoms predominantly in the upper airways. Some papers describing this have already been discussed.[43,44] This irritant effect on the upper respiratory tract may be more than just a nuisance, occasionally being sufficiently severe to cause recurrent epistaxis (nose bleeds).[45] The ability to cause sensitisation, as with dermatitis, may also be relevant in provoking respiratory problems, in particular, asthma. Several cases of occupational asthma following exposure to glutaraldehyde have been reported, although they are infrequent, with only a few in the UK, and the amount and nature of exposure required to cause this effect is unclear. As with other sensitisers, very small doses, below the current UK exposure limits, may be sufficient to cause asthma in pre-sensitised subjects.[46,47]

Carcinogenicity

Glutaraldehyde is chemically related to formaldehyde, and not surprisingly questions have been raised about its possible carcinogenicity. Although glutaraldehyde readily reacts with proteins, it is less reactive with nucleic acids than formaldehyde in vitro, and is only weakly mutagenic, as judged by the Ames test.[48] No epidemiological evidence is available on the incidence of cancer in populations exposed to glutaraldehyde.

Exposure

Glutaraldehyde is less volatile than formaldehyde and so levels of exposure are lower than for formaldehyde. A study of skin and respiratory symptoms among hospital workers in two Swedish hospitals included some information on their exposure to this chemical.[49] Personal samples were collected over half-shift and short term 15 minute periods for both glutaraldehyde and formaldehyde, from workers performing cold disinfection of surgical instruments. Short term sampling found a geometric mean exposure of 0.012ppm (range <0.0025ppm-0.143ppm), and the half shift samples found a geometric mean exposure below the detection limit of the method used (<0.01ppm). Formaldehyde was not detected. The use of automatic processing techniques generally resulted in lower exposures than when staff used manual techniques. A study of workers in an endoscopy unit in a UK hospital in Newcastle upon Tyne reported the following exposures: personal sampler on theatre nurse 0.12ppm and static sample from a bench at the side of the endoscopy room 0.05ppm.[50] A recent paper on exposure to glutaraldehyde used in cold sterilisation and X ray processing confirmed that exposure of staff was in general below the current UK occupational exposure standard (OES).[51] The lowest range of concentrations of glutaraldehyde measured was 0.003-0.006 mg/m^3 for work in X ray development, and the highest, 0.014-0.13 mg/m^3, was encountered during the activation of glutaraldehyde, and emptying and filling tanks for cold sterilisation. Nevertheless, the authors concluded that it was not clear that the current OES represented a 'safe' exposure level, arguing that exposure of staff to glutaraldehyde could be further reduced.

There are no data on the possible environmental effects of glutaraldehyde outside the workplace, but because it is less used outside health care than formaldehyde, the contribution from the health care industry to any environmental effect is probably proportionately greater than for formaldehyde. Its potential for causing harm may well be less than that of formaldehyde but this has not been proven.

Ethylene oxide

Ethylene oxide is used as an intermediate in numerous industrial processes including the production of ethylene glycol (antifreeze) and non-ionic detergents; it is also a sterilant gas and fumigant. Although more than 2000 million kilos of ethylene oxide are produced annually in the USA, probably

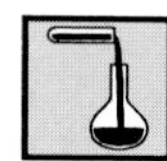

less than 1% of this is bought for medical or industrial sterilisation.[52] The IARC has estimated that in 1978 about 0.24% of annual US production of ethylene oxide was directed to health care, and in 1977 only 0.02% of total output directly from hospitals.[53] The small proportion in use for sterilisation may, however, represent an undue proportion of the total found in the environment, because much industrial use is either as an intermediate product, or in closed circuit processes. The UK authorities have set the official exposure limit for ethylene oxide at 5ppm.

The use of ethylene oxide in health care is more restricted than that of formaldehyde or glutaraldehyde. The chemical is most commonly found in units which are providing sterile supplies for an entire hospital or health district, and only relatively rarely is it found outside. The chemical acts as an irritant to the eyes, respiratory tract, and skin, and at high concentrations can cause depression of central nervous system activity.[54] In addition, ethylene oxide solutions can cause skin burns which may take between one and five hours to appear.

A survey of health care staff exposed to ethylene oxide found a statistically significant association between exposure and various symptoms that included eye irritation, skin irritation, skin rash, sore throat and shortness of breath.[55] Exposures to ethylene oxide were below the detection limit as an eight hour time-weighted average, although peak levels were recorded varying between 8.5ppm and 23.5ppm depending upon the type of steriliser. Symptoms were more common with sterilisers which produced higher peak exposures to ethylene oxide.

Persistent asthma after brief exposure to ethylene oxide in a patient with no previous history of chest disease has been reported.[56] The patient was not a health care worker, and the exposure was probably to quite high levels of ethylene oxide (>700ppm) which would not be encountered during normal sterilising procedures.

Exposure to ethylene oxide has been associated with some neurological effects in a few individuals, the symptoms described being weakness, foot drop, and dysaesthesia (abnormalities of sensation).[57,58] Biopsy findings showed axonal degeneration with secondary demyelination of the nerves.

Carcinogenicity

Several studies have shown that ethylene oxide is both mutagenic and carcinogenic in animals.[59] The evidence in humans is conflicting with some studies suggesting an above average incidence of leukaemia and stomach cancer.[60] Other studies, however, did not report any association between exposure and disease. A recent epidemiological study of 2,876 workers in the UK exposed to ethylene oxide (virtually all the exposed population) showed slightly raised, but statistically insignificant, total mortality rates from cancer, and no above average rates from cancers previously associated with exposure, namely, leukaemia and stomach cancer.[61] The authors concluded, "levels of exposure, although lower than in cohorts reported

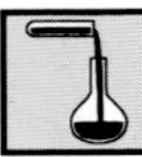

from Sweden, will have been higher than those found in industry today. Our findings do not exclude the possibility that ethylene oxide is a human carcinogen, particularly at higher exposures, but when viewed in the context of other published epidemiological studies, they suggest that any risk of cancer from currently permitted exposures is small". The IARC has recently argued that while there was sufficient evidence to conclude that ethylene oxide was an animal carcinogen there was only limited evidence that it was carcinogenic in humans.[62]

Exposure

Several papers have described exposure to ethylene oxide among hospital staff. One paper looked at 12 American hospitals believed by the investigators to use sterilisers and aerators representative of the standard types found in all hospitals.[63] Using personal samplers, the investigators found eight hour time-weighted average exposures ranged from "not detected" to 6.3ppm for "steriliser operators", and "not detected" to 6.7ppm for "packers and folders". Peak short term exposures ranged from "not detected" to 103.0ppm for the "steriliser operators", but the figure for "packers and folders" was not given. Unfortunately neither this paper, nor another which seemed to be based on the same data, included sufficient detail to allow a more thorough examination of exposure effects.[64] Both these papers did show, however, that employees at those hospitals with the best engineering controls and work practices did have the lowest mean exposure, suggesting that these measures were beneficial.

Another study was based on both area sampling and personal sampling from 104 workers at 12 hospitals in Canada.[65] Ambient samples from the work area around the sterilisers showed no detectable concentrations of ethylene oxide in any of the hospitals. The personal samples showed an eight hour time-weighted average exposure below the detection limit, with short term exposure (the duration of a single sterilisation cycle) ranging from "not detected" to 10.7ppm, with a mean value of 3.4ppm. The highest exposures occurred when the steriliser door was opened. Peak values then were 23.5ppm for portable sterilisers, 11.0ppm for a table top steriliser, and 8.5ppm for a built-in steriliser. These values, however, were only short lived, the levels of ethylene oxide dropping to less than 1ppm within a minute for the portable and table top sterilisers. Although these peak levels may represent a low overall exposure, as reflected in the eight hour time weighted average values, they cannot be dismissed as inconsequential as they may be important in the aetiology of some adverse effects.

Staff remote from the steriliser who may be exposed when opening sterilised packs of surgical instruments, etc, may be at theoretical risk of exposure. One paper has reported results of samples taken in an operating theatre as packs of surgical instruments were opened.[66] None of the samples collected were above the detection limit of ethylene oxide, which for the method used was approximately 0.02ppm.

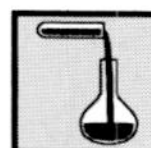

Methyl methacrylate

Methyl methacrylate is a constituent in the production of acrylic sheet and acrylic mouldings as well as inks and adhesives. In the health care sector exposure rarely occurs in isolation, but usually in operating theatres or dental laboratories where staff may also be exposed to anaesthetic gases and other chemicals. Because of this, little data is available on the possible effects of exposure to methyl methacrylate on health care staff. Methyl methacrylate is an irritant of the eyes, skin, and mucous membranes at concentration of 170-250ppm, with concentrations of 2300ppm being unbearable.[67] Headache, irritability, pain in the extremities, loss of memory, excessive fatigue, and sleep disturbances have all been reported.[68] Staff handling methyl methacrylate have been reported to develop sensory abnormalities, but these have not been reported in subjects exposed only to the vapour.[69] The current UK exposure limit is 100ppm (eight hour time-weighted average values) or 125ppm (10 minute short time exposure limit).

Studies have identified sensitisation to acrylates, including methyl methacrylate, and the subsequent development of allergic dermatitis and asthma.[70,71] There is little published information on the possible carcinogenic effects of exposure to methyl methacrylate, and the IARC concluded that data on human and animal carcinogenicity were inadequate.[72]

Exposure

Canadian researchers have reported on exposure to methyl methacrylate in a study assessing the exposure of operating room personnel to various potentially harmful agents.[73] Twenty seven personal samples were collected from orthopaedic operating theatres in which methyl methacrylate bone cement was being used. Only four samples gave values above the detection limit of 0.3ppm, these values being 0.9ppm, 1.0ppm, 1.0ppm, and 13.5ppm. Again, although the average exposure over a full shift might have been low, intermittent high peaks cannot be dismissed as inconsequential since they may be important in producing some adverse effects.

Darkroom disease

Staff working in diagnostic x-ray departments may also suffer adverse health effects from exposure to fumes released during processing of films. The health effects of exposure to processing fumes result from sensitisation to one or more chemicals contained in the fumes and are collectively known as ‘darkroom disease’. X-ray film processing fumes are covered by the COSHH regulations which require managers to carry out detailed and comprehensive assessments, and to prevent or control occupational exposure. The Department of Health also issues guidance recommending the effective control of x-ray film processing fumes. A report from the Society of Radiographers made a number of recommendations for the prevention of darkroom disease including the production of legally enforceable guidance on safety, improved internal exhaust systems in processing equipment and the provision of lower toxicity chemicals.[74]

Therapeutic drugs as chemicals

Many chemicals are regularly used in the health care sector because they are biologically active, and staff may be exposed to these chemicals in various ways. In addition, some of these chemicals will be metabolised and excreted after administration to patients, and will eventually be discharged with waste from the patient's residence or the hospital.

Several agents used therapeutically are recognised as sensitisers and as prescribed causes of occupational asthma in the UK, including antibiotics, cimetidine, ispaghula, and ipecacuanha.[75] In specific occupations the development of certain health conditions resulting from the use of these agents qualifies the sufferer for industrial injuries disablement benefit. In general, the pharmaceutical industry recognises these problems and has instituted control measures to prevent occupational exposure of employees. Relatively little work has been published on morbidity and mortality among health care workers other than doctors and so any risk encountered by employees when working with sensitising agents is difficult to estimate.

In addition to the sensitising agents used in health care, concern has also arisen over cytotoxic drugs used to treat malignant disease. These agents comprise a large proportion of IARC class I carcinogens (ie, the agent is carcinogenic to humans). Although most evidence has arisen in subjects treated with these agents rather than those exposed occupationally, there is clearly some potential for harm among those occupationally exposed and some evidence that this happens. An increase in markers of genetic damage (sister chromatid exchange in lymphocytes) has been described among nurses regularly handling cytostatic agents.[76] Unfortunately, the full implications of these findings, if any, has still to be established because the relevance of these abnormalities as meaningful markers of genetic damage is unclear. Theoretically, some of these drugs could retain some activity even after they have been used therapeutically and excreted, but the amounts and concentrations discharged in this way are likely to be small and probably create little risk of adverse effects. Nevertheless, it may be that a better way of disposing of these chemicals can be found rather than simply diluting them within the environment.

Discussion

Clearly it would be impracticable to abandon the use of chemicals in the health care sector. It would therefore be sensible to try and limit their use so as to prevent or lessen any adverse effects they may have, both to workers occupationally exposed and to the environment outside the workplace. Attempts to do this, however, are handicapped by a dearth of information. Even for the four widely used chemicals discussed in this chapter, it has

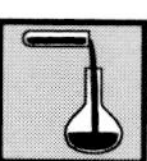

been difficult to find accurate information on the quantity used within the health service. Levels of workplace contamination by these same four chemicals have not been well investigated. NHS staff exposed to these and other chemicals may represent an undue proportion of all those at risk since industrial processes are more easily automated than health care, and industry tends to be more rigorous than the health service in controlling people's exposure to chemicals. The factors that may effect exposure in the workplace are poorly characterised, and although a risk assessment of exposures possibly hazardous to health is required by law, few hospitals have access to occupational hygiene services to conduct exposure assessments. We lack knowledge of exposures to other chemicals in the workplace and information is scarce about environmental contamination outside the workplace by these chemicals.

If information on exposure is difficult to come by, so too is information on possible adverse effects. For instance, we are not sure whether formaldehyde, probably the most comprehensively investigated of these chemicals, is carcinogenic or not. Nor do we know what levels of exposure are required to cause the other well proven adverse effects. Toxicological evidence in humans is limited, and extrapolation from animal or other research is fraught with difficulties (see Chapter 2 Environmental toxicology). Several chemicals are carcinogenic to one animal species but not to another. For most of the other chemicals in the health care sector possible adverse effects are, if anything, less well characterised. The precise concentrations and pattern of exposure required to cause the known adverse effects cannot generally be accurately measured.

Even with the limited evidence available we can reasonably assume that exposures are sufficient to cause adverse effects in some health care workers. Less easy to estimate are the numbers who may be affected. Irritant symptoms will occur in different individuals at different levels of exposure. Some of the adverse effects described depend upon the development of prior sensitisation. This is true for allergic dermatitis and asthma in particular, and the processes underlying this are not understood. We do know, however, that once sensitisation has developed otherwise trivial exposures may be sufficient to precipitate marked symptoms. We may reasonably estimate that the risk of occupational illnesses arising from the chemicals used in health care is relatively small compared with the risks generated in other industries. To be confident about this, however, we need much more information, including large epidemiological studies of workers in the health care and other sectors.

Epidemiological studies, particularly of cancer, are notoriously difficult to organise and interpret, and may take many years to produce results. One way of attempting to identify the long term or chronic effects of occupational exposures of chemicals on health is by studying the different groups of people who are exposed to them in health care. Much time and money will be needed to research fully the question of the possible adverse impact of chemicals used in the health service. Employers already have a legal duty under COSHH to assess the risks to the health of their employees arising from a number of sources, including chemicals, and for sensitising agents COSHH requires health monitoring of exposed staff. Occupational health physicians have a key role to play in carrying out such monitoring, keeping detailed information by specialty on occupation-related illness, including confirmation of adverse effects resulting from chemical exposures. The NHS Research and Development Directorate should review the need for research into occupational and environmental problems associated with the use of chemicals in the health care sector and establish a central database of research in this area. With such information it should be possible to make a fuller and more valid assessment of the possible effects to individuals, workers and the environment of chemicals used in providing health care.

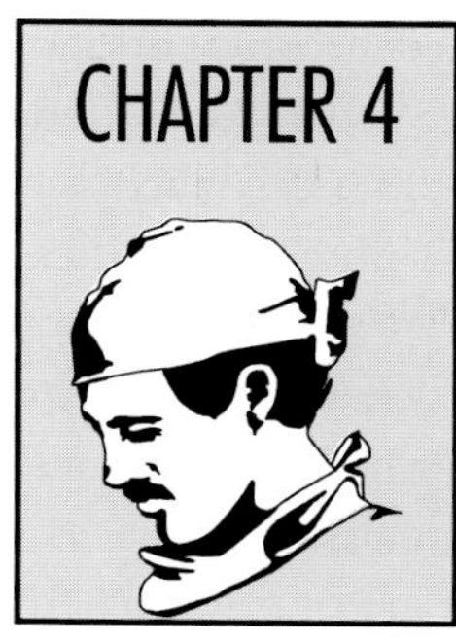

Waste anaesthetic gases

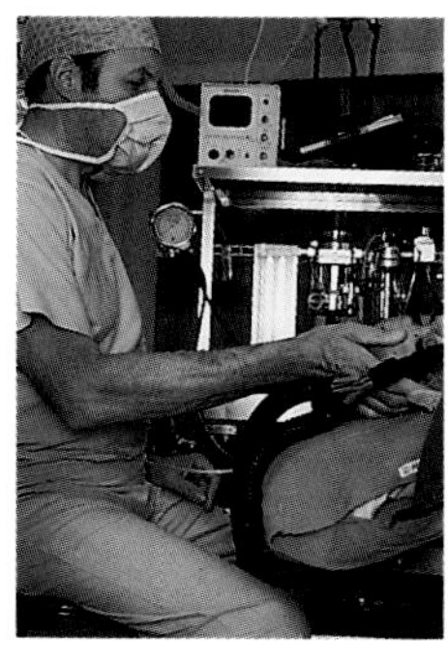

Anaesthetists and operating theatre staff should not be exposed to waste anaesthetic gases

Since the end of the 19th century, evidence has accumulated on the harmful effects of anaesthetic gases. Studies in the 1970s heightened concern over the health of anaesthetists. Several studies have assessed the possible adverse effects of anaesthetic agents among operating theatre staff, in obstetric units during childbirth, in dentistry, and in other settings in the health sector. Such has been the concern that in many settings where anaesthetic gases are used scavenging systems collect waste gas so that staff are not unduly exposed. This waste, however, must still be disposed of safely, and this has created further problems as communities and governments have become more worried about the environment. The Environmental Protection Act (1990) reflects this increasing concern about waste disposal, reinforcing the concept that the 'polluter pays'. It introduced new responsibilities under the general principle that those disposing of waste should use the 'best available technology not entailing excessive cost' (BATNEEC) to achieve the best practicable environmental option. It also introduces a requirement for licensing and documentation of each step in waste disposal. So simply venting waste anaesthetic gases to the environment may fail to meet the challenge of BATNEEC and does not represent the best practicable environmental option.

This chapter reviews the use of anaesthetic agents, considers the evidence of possible exposure levels and adverse effects among health care workers and examines published evidence of the possible effects of waste anaesthetic gas emissions upon the wider environment.

How anaesthetic gases are used

Anaesthetic gases may be divided broadly into two groups. The first is nitrous oxide, which is still widely used for its analgesic as well as its anaesthetic properties. The second encompasses the volatile halogenated hydrocarbons such as halothane, isoflurane, and enflurane, which have largely replaced ether and chloroform. Most operating theatres will contain equipment for delivering a combination of some or all of these agents to patients. Usually a mixture of nitrous oxide and one of the halogenated hydrocarbons is used to produce a good combination of anaesthesia and analgesia.

Anaesthetic machines deliver accurately measured concentrations of nitrous oxide mixed with oxygen, and by bubbling this gas through a vaporiser chamber vapours of the volatile hydrocarbon agents can be added in the correct concentration. Nitrous oxide and oxygen are usually delivered from a high pressure source and the pressure reduced within the machine. The volatile hydrocarbon agents are normally supplied as liquids in bottles which are used to top up the vaporiser on the machine as appropriate.

Anaesthetics may be used in either an open or closed system, or a system somewhere between these two. An open system is one in which the patient's exhaled breath is wasted complete with unused anaesthetic gases, nowadays by ducting outside the operating theatre. A closed or semi closed system is one in which all or some of the exhaled breath is recirculated to the patient after appropriate adjustment of oxygen and carbon dioxide concentrations, so more efficiently using anaesthetic gases. Many operating theatres are now designed to ensure good overall ventilation, and they incorporate scavenging equipment intended to collect exhaled and leaked anaesthetic gases so that unduly high concentrations do not accumulate within the operating theatre. In the case of day surgery, where a patient is admitted for investigation or operation on a planned non-resident basis with recovery facilities, the design specification and equipment of the anaesthetic room is identical to those of the normal in-patient equivalent. Because of its short-stay nature, day surgery requires the highest anaesthetic standards.[1] The longer the operation, the more general anaesthetic sedation or local anaesthetic is required. As new drugs are developed, more rapid recovery times can be expected. Nevertheless, gas-scavenging devices are an essential requirement in order to minimise the risk of exposure to waste anaesthetic gases.

Anaesthetic gases may enter the operating theatre environment from various sources. Hoses and other equipment sometimes leak during normal

Exposure to waste anaesthetic gases

Patients' exhaled breath may cause substantial contamination of operating theatres, particularly in unscavenged areas —

- when these exhalations may not be ducted out of the room;
- when a facial mask is used rather than an endotracheal tube, such as during induction;
- when a series of short operations is done;
- during paediatric surgery, because of the design of equipment used in paediatric anaesthesia.[2]

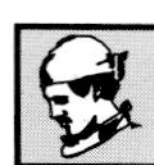

use, particularly at connections in the high pressure part of the system, or from spills when staff are filling vaporisers (see box on page 42).

Leaks may also occur from equipment if it is left switched on when not in use by the patient - for example, when a patient is intubated during induction of anaesthesia the mask may be put on one side for a few seconds with the gas flow still on. Although operating theatres are now normally scavenged, fewer recovery rooms and ward areas are so equipped. Since patients may absorb large amounts of fat soluble anaesthetic agents during anaesthesia and exhale them as they recover, substantial contamination of these areas may occur. As these agents are fat soluble some leakage may also theoretically occur from surgical wounds.

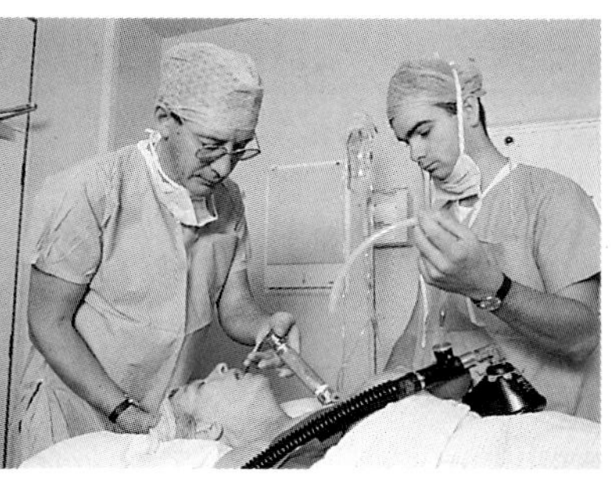

During induction of anaesthesia and manipulation of the mask, gas may leak into the operating theatre environment

Anaesthetic agents are not just used in the well controlled environment of a hospital operating theatre but in many settings throughout the health sector. Nitrous oxide is a constituent of 'entonox', widely used for its analgesic properties in ambulances, during childbirth in the delivery rooms of maternity hospitals, and in a host of other places such as on general hospital wards during painful procedures, and in first aid rooms in the workplace for use in the event of an accident. Few of these places will have any scavenging equipment to collect and vent waste gases. Anaesthetic agents are also widely used in dentistry, where they may have to be given by a nasal route. This mode of delivery is more prone to leakage than via an endotracheal tube or orinasal mask, and where scavenging equipment is rarely used. Some dentists also use nitrous oxide for its analgesic and sedative effects on patients.

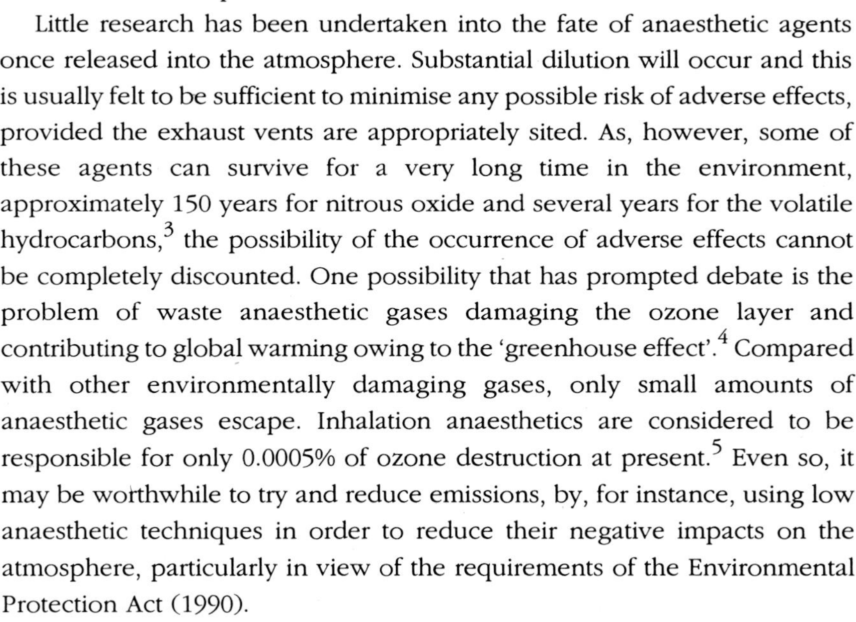

Little research has been undertaken into the fate of anaesthetic agents once released into the atmosphere. Substantial dilution will occur and this is usually felt to be sufficient to minimise any possible risk of adverse effects, provided the exhaust vents are appropriately sited. As, however, some of these agents can survive for a very long time in the environment, approximately 150 years for nitrous oxide and several years for the volatile hydrocarbons,[3] the possibility of the occurrence of adverse effects cannot be completely discounted. One possibility that has prompted debate is the problem of waste anaesthetic gases damaging the ozone layer and contributing to global warming owing to the 'greenhouse effect'.[4] Compared with other environmentally damaging gases, only small amounts of anaesthetic gases escape. Inhalation anaesthetics are considered to be responsible for only 0.0005% of ozone destruction at present.[5] Even so, it may be worthwhile to try and reduce emissions, by, for instance, using low anaesthetic techniques in order to reduce their negative impacts on the atmosphere, particularly in view of the requirements of the Environmental Protection Act (1990).

Levels of exposure to anaesthetic gases

Exposure to anaesthetic gases may vary widely depending on many factors, such as the type of operation, anaesthetic technique used, and the setting in which they are used. Occupational exposure limits for these agents have been set in the UK only from 1 January 1994, although other countries have had exposure limits for longer periods[6] (Table 4.1).

Table 4.1
UK occupational exposure standards to anaesthetic gases

Agent	*Occupational Exposure Standards (8 hour time-weighted average) (ppm)*
Nitrous oxide	100
Halothane	10
Enflurane	20
Isoflurante	50

Source: Health and Safety Executive. Occupational Exposure Limits. EH40-1994

Operating theatres

Several studies have estimated exposure of health service staff to anaesthetic agents, but only a few have used personal sampling to measure individual exposure during operating sessions rather than area sampling. One study that did use personal samples estimated the exposure of a group of anaesthetists administrating a variety of anaesthetic gases, techniques and equipment, but without scavenging. Samples were collected during a three hour operating session, thus representing an average exposure during various activities. The mean exposure to nitrous oxide was determined to be 269ppm (range 108-430ppm), and to halothane to be 3.6ppm (range 1-8ppm).[7] The same study also included several anaesthetic sessions in an operating theatre with scavenging equipment and the mean exposure here to nitrous oxide was 127ppm (range 67.5-225ppm) and to halothane 0.57ppm (range 0-1.6ppm).

A study of an operating theatre in a Birmingham teaching hospital sampled air from several sites approximating to the breathing zones for surgeons and other operating theatre staff.[8] The median concentrations of halothane were 55.7ppm in the theatre, when unscavenged and 19.7ppm when scavenged. Although the scavenging system reduced median contamination overall, a significant reduction was not seen at all sites because the ventilation arrangements varied. This study did not report the concentrations of nitrous oxide.

Several other studies have reported contamination levels of operating theatres and adjacent rooms used for induction of anaesthesia, recovery, etc. These are summarised in table 4.2, with the results mainly given as an average exposure during an eight hour working period which should not be exceeded. These results show considerable exposure, often above the standards adopted in other countries. The concentration of waste anaesthetic gases in an operating theatre may not be the same as that to which theatre workers are exposed since they often spend time working outside the theatre. Only those studies incorporating personal sampling accurately

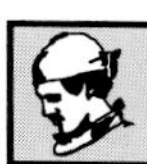

Table 4.2: Reports of average anaesthetic gas contamination

*Reference** (*For full details see chapter reference list)	*Room in which sample collected*	*Scavenging*	*Nitrous oxide ppm*	Halothane ppm
Davenport et al 1976[9]	anaesthetist	no	269	3.6
	personal sample	yes	127	0.57
	operating theatre	no	453	5.3
	operating theatre	yes	62	0.46
	induction room	no	3038	52.1
	induction room	yes	152	3.1
Davenport et al 1980[10]	induction room	no	187	1.9
	operating theatre			
	periphery	no	171	1.3
	by anaesthetist	no	189	2.0
	anaesthetist (personal)	no	381	3.1
	recovery room	no	30	0.43
Thompson et al 1981[11]	operating theatre	no		55.7 (449µg/1)
	operating theatre	yes		19.7 (159µg/1)
Boyland 1982[12]	operating theatre	yes	peak >570	
	recovery room	no	peak >600	2.0 (peak >5.8)
Thompson et al 1987[13]	operating theatre (anaesthetist)			
	poorly ventilated	unclear	365 (656mg/m^3)	23.7 (191.3mg/m^3)
	well ventilated	unclear	218 (392mg/m^3)	4.4 (35.6mg/m^3)
	operating theatre (operating dept assist)			
	poorly ventilated	unclear	110 (197mg/m^3)	6.3 (50.7mg/m^3)
	well ventilated	unclear	72 (129mg/m^3)	2.4 (19.7mg/m^3)
Gray 1989[14]	operating theatre	yes	range 3 - 5120	
Gardner 1989[15]	operating theatre	no	94	1.7
		yes	32	0.7
	recovery room	no	27	0.6
Rajhans et al 1989[16]	operating theatre	almost always	37.6	0.07
	recovery room	unclear	28.7	
Sass-Kortsak et al 1992[17]	operating theatre (anaesthetist)	yes	10	
	operating theatre (nurse)		5.4	

reflect exposure, others give a guide only to possible maximum exposure. In addition, although scavenging and general ventilation reduce average levels of exposure, they cannot be assumed to remove all waste gases.

The results in table 4.2 show average exposure to waste anaesthetic gases within operating theatres. Several of these studies have suggested that not all groups working in operating theatres may be equally exposed. Thompson et al,[18] in a study using personal sampling throughout a half day operating session, found that average exposure level fell in the following order: anaesthetist, surgeon, scrub nurse, other nurse, operating department assistant (ODA), nursing auxiliary. Median exposure to nitrous oxide of the anaesthetists during the half day operating session was more than four times that for the nursing auxiliaries (321ppm and 69ppm respectively), while for halothane the differences were greater (23ppm and 3ppm). Unsurprisingly, subsequent studies have confirmed that anaesthetists are usually exposed to higher average levels of waste anaesthetic gases than others working in the operating theatre.[19-22] Episodes of exposure where levels above those standards shown in table 4.1 are encountered are also more frequent for anaesthetists than for any other group.

Obstetrics

Although anaesthetic gases are widely used in obstetric care, few studies have documented exposure outside operating theatres. One study measured the exposure of midwives to nitrous oxide using personal samplers and averaging levels of exposure across the duration of the shift for which the sampler was worn (a mean duration of between six hours 18 minutes and seven hours 54 minutes depending upon hospital).[23] Midwives working in the delivery rooms in four hospitals took part. The half oxygen, half nitrous oxide (entonox) gas mix was used in all hospitals, but only one hospital used any scavenging system. Mean exposure varied from 41 to 363ppm. In three of the hospitals exposure concentrations averaged above 200ppm throughout a shift on several occasions, while in one, an average exposure of 400ppm across a shift was exceeded on some occasions.

Dental surgeries

Waste anaesthetic gases can also contaminate dental surgeries. General anaesthesia is used during conservation and extraction procedures, and nitrous oxide may also be given at other times for sedation and analgesia short of general anaesthesia. Measurements of the exposure of dentists to nitrous oxide have usually been rather higher than those in hospital operating theatres. One paper reported a mean exposure to nitrous oxide of dentists sampling from their breathing zone, during a session employing general anaesthesia, of 2445ppm (range 266-6281ppm).[24] These samples were collected without the use of scavenging equipment, as would be customary in dental surgeries. When scavenging was used mean exposure to nitrous oxide fell to 351ppm (range 92-1228ppm). Concentrations of nitrous oxide in the blood of dentists, and some of their assistants was also measured in this study and mean values were found to be higher for the dentists than the assistants (60.26 and 20.31 $\mu molN_2O/l$) and was further

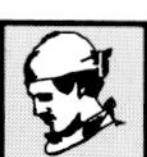

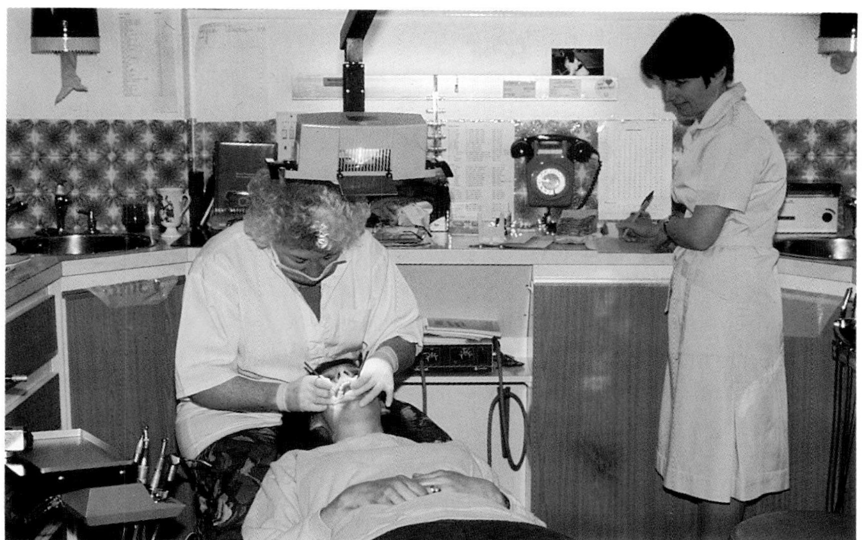

Waste anaesthetic gases can contaminate dental surgeries

reduced by scavenging (7.60 and 1.70 µmolN_2O/l). Clearly, the dentists were exposed to levels of waste nitrous oxide gas that were higher than the suggested limits shown in table 4.1. Exposure was lower for their assistants and was again effectively reduced by scavenging.

Environmental pollution

Although scavenging waste anaesthetic gases and exhausting them to the external atmosphere reduces contamination of the workplace environment, the possibility remains that this may be merely exchanging one problem for another. Potential hazards from exhausting waste anaesthetic gases to the environment have attracted attention, reflecting the community's heightened concern over environmental issues generally, and ozone-depleting and 'greenhouse' gases in particular. The volatile halogenated hydrocarbon anaesthetics, while not specifically included, have similar chemical structure to the fully halogenated chlorofluorocarbons regulated under the Montreal protocol, which seeks to stabilise and eventually to reduce their emission into the atmosphere. Estimates vary about the annual worldwide production of these agents. Most suggest that approximately 1,000 tonnes of halothane are produced yearly, as well as an estimated weight of between 1,000 and 5,400 tonnes of other agents such as isoflurane and enflurane.[25-27] Worldwide production of chlorofluorocarbons, the majority fully halogenated, probably exceeds 1,000,000 tonnes per year for use as refrigerants, propellants for aerosols, solvents, and foaming agents. Halogenated anaesthetic agents constitute only a small part of this total. Damage to the ozone layer depends not just upon quantity, however, but also upon the halogen content of the gas, which determines its reactivity with ozone, and its longevity and hence ability to reach the ozone layer. Most experts agree that the halogenated anaesthetic agents are less potent than the fully halogenated hydrocarbons in damaging the ozone layer, and that they are less long lived. So most estimates are that the damage they contribute to the ozone layer is considerably less than 1% of the total caused by this class of chemical.[28-31]

Nitrous oxide is recognised as a 'greenhouse' gas, reflecting heat back to the surface of the earth and so contributing to global warming. It may also indirectly contribute to ozone depletion. Medical use of nitrous oxide in the UK was approximately 1×10^9 litres in 1988, compared with an estimated production from other sources (microbial breakdown of agricultural nitrates, burning fossil fuels, etc) of approximately 8×10^9 to 3×10^{10} litres. Medical use therefore contributes only a fraction of the total nitrous oxide entering the atmosphere each year, although this may be a bigger proportionate contribution than that of the medical use of volatile halogenated hydrocarbon agents in the total use of chlorofluorocarbons.

Evidence of damage from waste anaesthetic gases

Known adverse effects

Anaesthetic gases affect the recipient's level of consciousness, behaviour, perception, and reasoning. These skills are important when performing complex tasks. The concentrations needed to induce anaesthesia are, however, much greater than are usually encountered during occupational or incidental exposures from atmospheric contamination. Nitrous oxide when used as an anaesthetic is usually given as a 50-70% mixture with oxygen (ie 500,000-700,000ppm), while halothane and the other volatile halogenated hydrocarbon agents are usually used at concentrations of 0.5-4% (ie 5,000-40,000ppm). Although there may be a small risk of these agents affecting the ability of operating theatre staff to perform their job, there is little evidence of this in practice. A recent review concluded, "present knowledge suggests that no acute behavioural alterations are produced by concentrations of nitrous oxide below 8-12% (80,000-120,000ppm) or by less than 0.1% (1,000ppm) of halothane".[32] Rather less is known of neuropsychiatric effects of chronic exposure to low levels of anaesthetic agents.[33,34]

Potential adverse effects of anaesthetic gases

- *Nitrous oxide:* Interference with the action of vitamin B_{12} (resulting in megaloblastic anaemia and possible neuropathy); depression of white cell formation
- *Halothane:* Severe hepatotoxicity although rare; (the risk seems to be increased by repeated exposures over a short period). Halogenated alkanes[35] may sensitise heart tissue to the effect of adrenergic stimulation
- *Enflurane and Isoflurane:* These gases have not been associated with severe hepatotoxicity, but there may be an immunogenic effect on hepatic tissue in susceptible subjects.

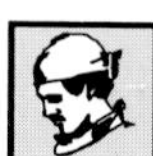

Several other adverse effects have been recognised both among patients who are given anaesthetic gases as part of their treatment and among those occupationally exposed. Although those working in an operating theatre, or exposed because of atmospheric contamination, will be exposed to much lower concentrations of gases than patients, there may, nonetheless, be a theoretical risk of staff experiencing adverse effects because their exposure will be of a longer duration. The British National Formulary[36] lists several of these, and other authoritative texts and articles have reviewed the possible adverse effects of these agents (see box on page 48). Casarett and Doull's *Toxicology* suggests that, "halothane induced hepatotoxicity can be considered as two entities. A mild form of liver injury is seen shortly after anaesthesia and can be reproduced in animals" (this may be similar to the injury that occurs following exposure to other halogenated hydrocarbons eg carbon tetrachloride, tetrachloroethane),"the other form, delayed and severe appears to be due to an immune-mediated mechanism. Patients with halothane-induced liver injury can generate liver antibodies that react with trifluoroacetyl-carrier proteins. There is also the suggestion that enflurane, as well as the trifluoroacetyl halide metabolite of halothane, covalently binds to similar hepatic proteins and may become immunogens in susceptible individuals".[37]

Nitrous oxide may cause a megaloblastic anaemia, neurological abnormalities, and damage to white blood cells, through an action on vitamin B_{12}.[38] Nitrous oxide can oxidise vitamin B_{12}, so interfering in the metabolism of methionine, folate, and thionine. Both a peripheral neuropathy and a condition similar to 'subacute combined degeneration', which is typical in vitamin B_{12} deficiency, have been reported among abusers of nitrous oxide. Nitrous oxide abusers of course, are likely to be exposed to higher levels of nitrous oxide than would commonly be encountered as a result of environmental contamination, or, among subjects who are occupationally exposed.[39,40]

There is evidence that halogenated alkanes as a group have effects on the heart. They are negatively chronotropic and inotropic at the concentration used for anaesthesia and sensitise the heart to the effect of adrenergic stimulation (possibly increasing the risk of arrhythmias).[41] Such stimulation may be encountered either physiologically during exercise or similar stimuli, or pharmacologically where adrenergic agents are used to treat asthma and similar conditions.

Concern has been raised that anaesthetic gases may cause damage to the foetus as a result of the exposure of pregnant women, these include fetotoxicity and teratogenicity. Other purported adverse effects include nephrotoxicity, and carcinogenicity. Although these effects, particularly the first two, have aroused much interest there has been less consensus about their relevance to those exposed as a result of workplace or more general atmospheric contamination. For most of these effects there have been either animal data suggesting an effect but difficulty in extrapolating the results to humans, or the available human evidence has in some way been inadequate or inconsistent.[42]

Mortality among those exposed to anaesthetic gases

Most of the available evidence suggests that anaesthetists are the most heavily exposed group working in an operating theatre (see Table 4.2). In addition, more data are available on the health of anaesthetists than other groups working with anaesthetic gases. Although anaesthetists have been more frequently exposed to organic solvents and other agents used as anaesthetic gases there appear to have been few recent studies of the mortality of anaesthetists within the UK since that of Doll and Peto in 1977.[43] This large study followed a cohort of 20,450 medical practitioners over 20 years and found a rise in the incidence of neoplasms of the pancreas among full time users of anaesthetic gases, but the rise was not statistically significant. No significant rise in other causes of mortality was found. Studies from the USA have not shown any additional cause of above average mortality rates, showing low all-cause mortality but high mortality from suicide, particularly among younger age groups.[44,45] In one study of 652 deaths among anaesthetists during 1947-71, 20% of all deaths among subjects aged 25 to 44 were the result of suicide, but it is difficult to attribute these to exposure to anaesthetic gases.[46] Harrington, however, in his review in 1987 concluded that, "to date, the published studies on anaesthetists do not suggest that the hazards of the operating room are translated into serious health risks for the staff who work there".[47]

Several effects which would not be reflected in mortality figures have been suggested and are relevant. It has been noted that exposure to anaesthetic agents may affect pregnancies. Knill-Jones et al surveyed 1,241 female anaesthetists and 1,678 female controls selected from the Medical Register.[48] Results were analysed by comparing anaesthetists who continued working during the first and second trimesters of pregnancy with those who did not, and control subjects. The anaesthetists who continued working had a higher incidence of congenital malformations among live births than those not working, but not higher than occurred among the controls. The working

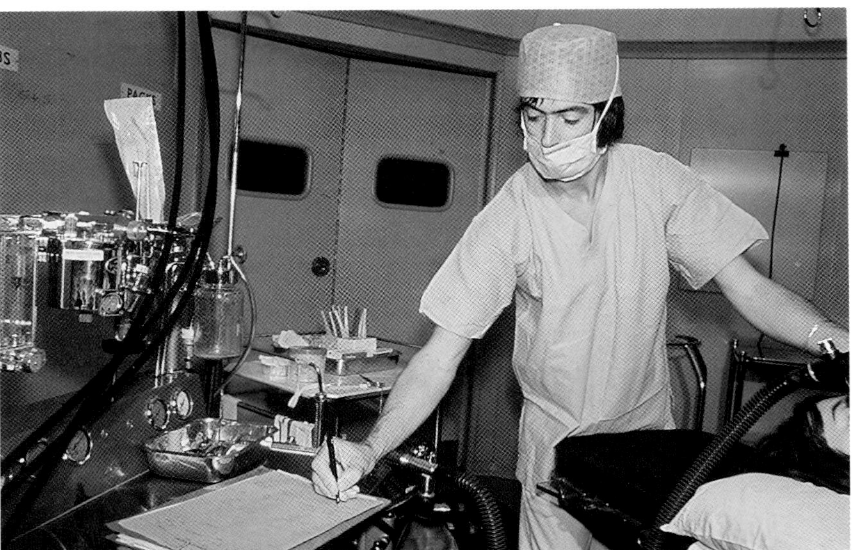

Anaesthetists are likely to be the occupational group most heavily exposed to waste anaesthetic gases

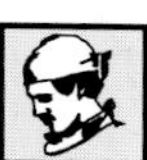

anaesthetists also had a higher incidence of spontaneous abortion than did the controls, but not higher than among the non working anaesthetists. So the message was unclear, and Harrington described the evidence on adverse outcome of pregnancy as, "flawed and subject to strong confounding and reporting bias".[49]

McNamee et al studied early retirement among anaesthetists and doctors in other medical specialties. The anaesthetists showed higher rates of retirement from ill health than the other groups.[50] A paper has also recently described a combination of neurophysiological symptoms occurring more commonly among anaesthetists working in poorly scavenged operating theatres than among those working in the best scavenged, or among control subjects.[51] Unfortunately, this study did not include any measurements of the actual exposures encountered in those operating theatres associated with symptoms and so the specific cause of these findings is not known.

Evidence of environmental effects of waste anaesthetic gases

Anaesthetic gases are produced in large amounts and used in many hospitals throughout the world. Almost all the gases used eventually find their way into the atmosphere, with very little being metabolised during use. As already observed, they form only a relatively small proportion of the total amount of 'greenhouse' and ozone depleting gases discharged to the atmosphere, so it is likely that their contribution to any such effect is small. In addition, several gases used in anaesthetic practice may have applications outside health care in the chemical industry, and so not all environmental contamination caused by their use is attributable to the health service. For anaesthetic agents other than nitrous oxide, there is little published evidence upon which to base an estimate of their use in industry. Nitrous oxide is, however, widely used outside health care, and the volatile halogenated hydrocarbon anaesthetic agents represent only a small proportion of the total halogenated hydrocarbons produced annually. So the relative contribution of health care to any environmental damage that may be caused by these agents is probably only a small proportion of that attributable overall to these agents.

Discussion

Although anaesthetic gases are widely used in medical care, they are known to have adverse effects on biological systems. These have usually been described following higher exposures than would be likely to result from environmental contamination of either the workplace or the external environment. Even so, the possibility remains that the levels of exposure encountered by those working in the health care industry could have adverse effects upon their nervous system, liver, kidney, haematological and reproductive systems. The available evidence on many of these issues is both conflicting and insufficient, and so it is hard to estimate whether a risk to health results from existing exposure levels, or if there is a level below which we can be confident that no adverse effect will occur. Consequently it would be prudent to restrict the exposure of those working with anaesthetic gases until sufficient evidence is available to make us confident that no ill effects are occurring.

At present the control of occupational exposure of those working with anaesthetic gases involves venting waste to the atmosphere, where their effect is largely unknown. But because of the large dilutions, and the fact these gases constitute only a small proportion of all possibly harmful waste released, we can reasonably assume the risk to the environment is small. Nevertheless, as the output of other harmful gases is controlled and reduced, waste anaesthetic gases may come to represent a larger proportion of agents potentially damaging to the environment. Furthermore, it could be argued that any damage to the environment should be avoided, even if it does only constitute a small proportion of the total. Legislation in the UK already requires the use of BATNEEC, and, if anything, will probably move towards more stringent control of waste in an effort to reduce environmental damage.

Control of anaesthetic gases in the workplace could be improved. The wider use of scavenging equipment, particularly where gases are used outside operating theatres, better designed leak proof equipment, and the development of anaesthetic techniques to reduce or eliminate waste, are possible. Furthermore, it is short sighted to vent waste gases to the atmosphere when it is possible to collect them onto adsorbent filters, collect, and reuse them. More research into the economical viability of collecting and reusing waste gases is needed. Appropriate equipment would have to be cheap and easy to use to ensure its wide adoption by 'small' users of anaesthetics such as dentists, who may nevertheless cumulatively contribute a large proportion of waste.

Some surgical and investigatory procedures now done using gas-induced general anaesthesia could well be done using local or regional anaesthesia, or intravenous general anaesthesia. These agents are usually given by injection, and are to a large extent metabolised and detoxified before being excreted from the body, so reducing their impact on the environment. For minor procedures which require local anaesthesia, complementary medicine techniques such as acupuncture and hypnosis might have a place if these are proved to be as effective as conventional techniques. This will require carefully controlled trials and assessment, but wider adoption of all these techniques could dramatically reduce the production of waste anaesthetic gases.

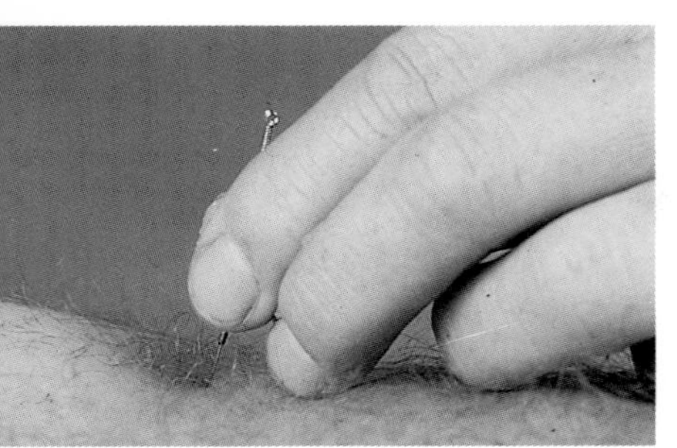

Acupuncture might have a place as an alternative to local anaesthesia for minor procedures

Changes in practice will require investment, either in equipment for collecting and recycling gases, or in research into alternative anaesthetic techniques. The widespread adoption of measures to reduce waste could save money, as well as cutting the risk of harm to patients, staff and the environment.

Ionising radiation

Radiation has always been present in the natural environment. Light and heat from the sun are natural forms of radiation that are essential to human existence. Other forms include radiowaves and microwaves for example. Radiation is often divided into two groups; ionising and non-ionising radiation, according to the effects it produces on matter. Non-ionising radiations include light, heat, radar, radiowaves, ultrasound and microwaves. Ionising radiation is emitted by elements in the earth's core or by material derived from these sources, as well as diagnostic and therapeutic x-ray machines and nuclear installations. Cosmic rays have an ionising component. Over the past century exposure to ionising radiation has gradually increased through medical, diagnostic and therapeutic practices, and during the past 50 years large amounts of radioactive substances have been utilised for a variety of other purposes.

The National Radiological Protection Board estimates that the average person in Britain receives an ionising radiation dose of 2.6mSv each year.[1] Of this, 85.5% comes from natural sources, 14% from medical radiation practices and 0.5% from other man-made sources such as discharges from nuclear installations. However, exposure is not distributed evenly through the population, and some individuals will have lower or higher exposure than average. (Figure 5.1)

The average dose rates from the ionising component of cosmic radiation increases with altitude and latitude. Exposure to cosmic rays therefore increases during air travel, and the dose received depends on the route taken and the overall distance flown. Frequent fliers (who spend perhaps 100 hours in flight during the year) would receive a dose of 400μSv. A dose approaching 1mSv could be received if the flights were on transpolar routes, eg 5 flights from UK to Japan. With the exception of radon, where measures are possible to reduce levels of radon gas in homes, exposure to other

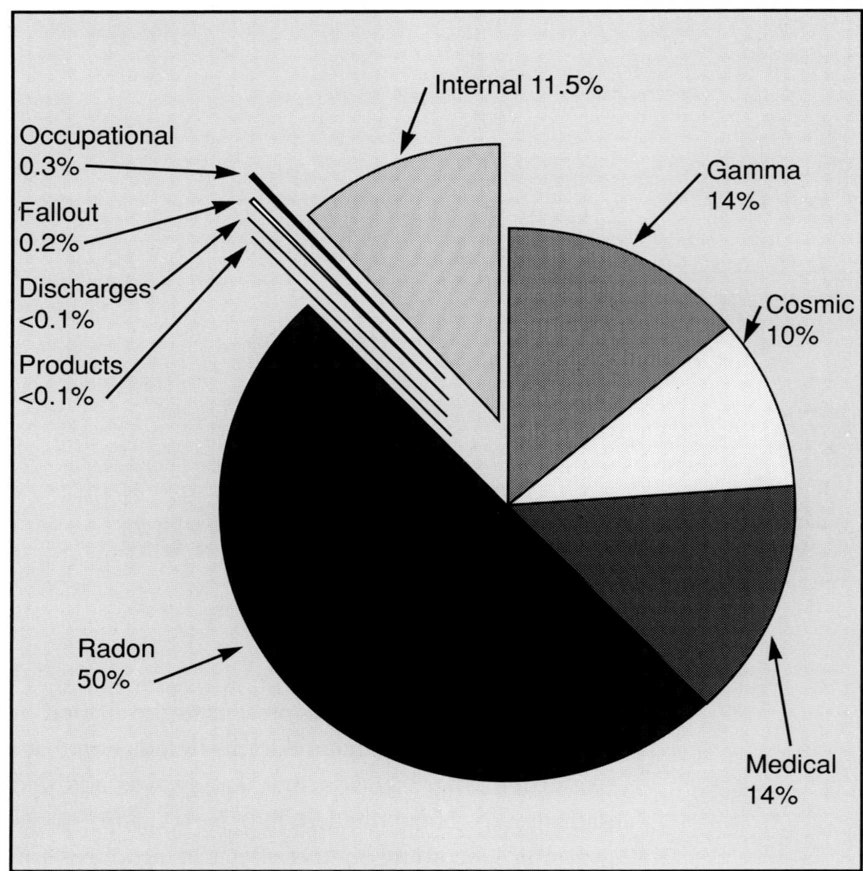

Figure 5.1: Average annual radiation dose to the UK population

natural sources cannot be changed. Individual annual doses of radon can range between 100μSv and 100,000μSv a year. Higher levels of radiation are associated with granite rocks, such as in the far south-west of England.[2] (Figure 5.2) The UK population receives an average annual dose of radiation from all natural sources of 2210μSv. With regard to medical sources, it is important to note that not everyone receives an x-ray examination or treatment in a particular year. It has been estimated that for diagnostic radiology well over half the population has no x-ray examinations during a given year.[3]

Radiation does have the potential to affect our environment, and in this chapter we examine how as a result of a combination of physical and chemical properties radiation used in medical practice can affect both human and other biological systems both inside and outside the hospital.

Radioactivity and radiation

When radiation passes through matter, including tissue, it deposits some of its energy in the material concerned as a result of interactions with both atomic nuclei and electrons. Charged alpha and beta particles deposit energy as a result of interactions with the electrons in the proximity of their path. Gamma rays and x-rays deposit energy in a variety of ways involving the

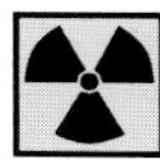

to radiation in the vicinity of its source. The ions produced when ionising radiations interact with atoms in materials are chemically active and react with proteins and other tissue constituents to produce biological effects. (Figure 5.3)

Ionisation may occur extensively along the transmission path through the material. The intensity of the chemical reaction, and therefore the likelihood of a biological effect, increases with the density of ionisation at a point. Alpha particles and neutrons lead to dense ionisation and have a high linear energy transfer (LET), while x-rays, gamma rays and high energy electrons produce a less dense ionisation, albeit often penetrating further into tissues, and have a lower LET.

The biological effects of exposure of a tissue to ionising radiation depend both upon the site within a cell in which the ionisation and consequent chemical change occurs, and the number of such ionisations within a cell. The changes provoked in a cell may range from minor repairable impairment of its function to death. Changes in one cell may affect the functioning of adjacent cells, and therefore the tissue or organ consisting of these cells, and consequently may even affect the whole organism. In humans and other animals the biological effects of radiation may be either somatic or genetic. Somatic changes include 'burning' and scarring which results from the functional impairment in cells or tissues, and may be progressive over months or years. Although the ways in which radiation damages cells are not fully understood, many involve changes to the deoxyribonucleic acid (DNA). Such chemical changes may have a harmful biological effect, leading to genetic changes. This may lead to the development of malignant tumours or to inherited genetic defects in the descendants of people who have been exposed to radiation. Leukaemia and solid tissue cancers may take several decades to develop after radiation damage.

Measuring exposure

The dose of radiation received by people or things is measured in terms of grays (Gy). It is possible to calculate the dose absorbed by an organ if the activity in it is known. This absorbed dose is the quantity of energy imparted by ionising radiation to a unit mass of matter, such as tissue. Equal absorbed doses do not necessarily have equal biological effects: 1 gray of alpha radiation is more harmful to tissue than 1 gray of beta radiation, because an alpha particle, being slower and more heavily charged, loses its energy more densely along its path in tissue. The relative biological effectiveness (RBE) is therefore used to put all ionising radiations on an equal basis with regard to their potential for causing harm. The equivalent (absorbed dose multiplied by RBE) is expressed in sieverts (Sv). For gamma rays, x-rays, and beta particles the RBE is set at 1. For alpha particles, it is set at 20, ie a dose of 1 Gy of alpha radiation corresponds to a dose equivalent of 20Sv. This provides an index of the risk of harm from exposure to various radiations irrespective of their type of energy.

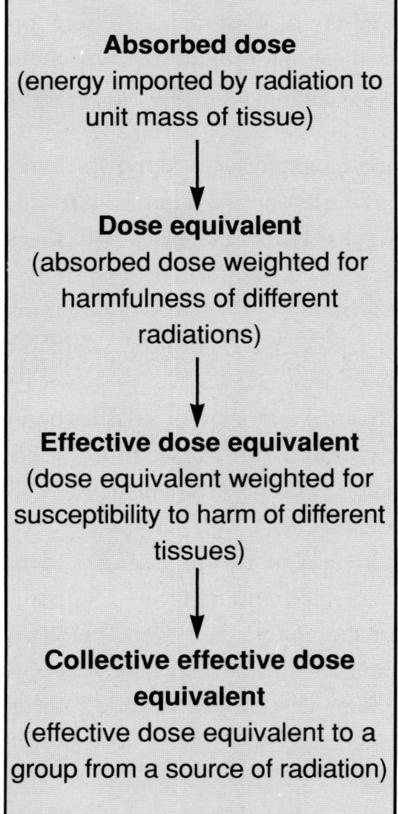

Figure 5.4: Measuring exposure to ionising radiation

The risk of fatal malignancy per Sv is not the same for various tissues of the body, and the risk of serious hereditary damage, through irradiating the testes and ovaries must also be taken into account. The dose equivalents in each of the major organs and tissues are therefore weighted in relation to the risk associated with that particular organ. The effective dose equivalent is used to provide a broad indicator to health from any exposure to ionising radiation irrespective of the type and energy of the radiation, whether internal or external, taking into account the susceptibility to harm of different tissues. It is often useful to have a measure of the total radiation dose to which a group of people or a whole population are exposed. The quantity used to express this total is the collective effective dose equivalent. This is obtained by adding, over all groups in the population, the product of the average effective dose equivalent to the group from the source being considered and the number of people in that group[5] (Figure 5.4).

Sources of medical ionising radiation

Ionising radiations cannot be detected by any of the human senses. Except when a person receives a very high dose, (eg in a major industrial nuclear incident or in nuclear warfare) there are no immediate effects. Widespread ignorance and fear exist about the possible effects of exposure to even small amounts of radiation, often unjustifiably. This fear is not confined to the public, doctors who have no reason in their normal practice to be familiar with the effects of ionising radiation may also be unduly alarmed. Some techniques in medical practice such as diathermy, ultrasound and magnetic resonance imaging use non-ionising radiation, while others such as computed tomography involve relatively large exposures of ionising radiation. Not everyone understands the distinction between the two types and different doses involved.

The sources of ionising radiation used in medicine may be either from radioactive substances or 'x-ray machines'. Initially the radioactive substances used in health care were naturally occurring ones such as radium, but nowadays artificially produced radio-isotopes are almost always used. The quality and quantity of radiation produced by isotopes depends on the

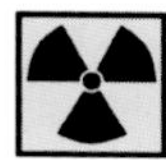

isotope source and so varies greatly in energy and penetrating power. Similarly, 'x-ray machines' may produce x-rays, electrons or other charged particles; each may be produced with a wide range of different energy levels depending on the design of the apparatus. A wide choice of possible sources therefore exists to produce the type of ionising radiation which is required for a particular patient, but with the potential for producing effects in the wider environment.

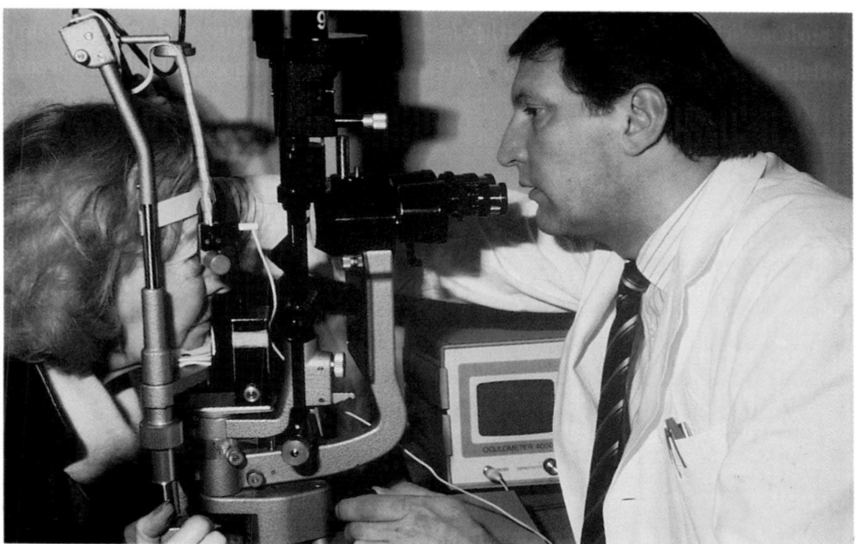

Ultrasound scanning equipment uses non-ionising radiation

Diagnostic x-ray machines

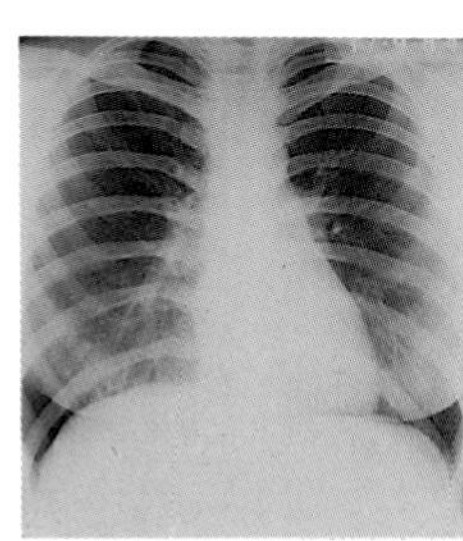

Radiograph of a normal female chest produced by a diagnostic x-ray machine

Diagnostic x-ray machines are mostly found located within radiology departments of hospitals. They work at relatively low energies of up to approximately 200keV (kilo electron Volts) and invariably have some safety mechanisms incorporated in their design, for example, a thick casing made of an element with a high atomic number, such as lead. Additionally, the siting of the machines and the construction of the rooms are designed to promote safe working.[6] Strict operating rules and regular monitoring of exposure to staff ensure that working practices are safe. In accordance with the Ionising Radiation Regulations (1985) Approved Code of Practice,[7] investigations are carried out if an individual employee's cumulative radiation dose during a five year period, exceeds 75mSv.[8] Fortunately, monitoring only rarely shows significant unwanted exposure. Diagnostic x-ray machines are also used in other parts of hospitals, for example, portable ones for examinations in wards, operating theatres, etc. In such locations, protection arrangements may be less satisfactory and strict operating rules less easy to implement and monitor. While the staff of x-ray departments are trained to meet the safety requirements of radiological practice, the use of diagnostic x-ray apparatus elsewhere may not always be controlled by trained radiologists or radiographers. Diagnostic x-ray machines may also be used in GPs' surgeries, during domiciliary consultations, or for mobile screening in vehicles. Mobile screening units such as modern breast screening units must comply with all safety requirements.

Computed tomography

Computed tomography (CT) is an x-ray imaging technique providing excellent radiographic contrast between soft tissues providing high-quality clinical information for localised planes within the body. CT has proliferated steadily in the UK over the last 20 years to form an integral part of medical radiology. The excellence of CT images has undoubtedly led to significant advances in patient care, and has replaced many other often more invasive diagnostic techniques, which presented risks to the patient such as from an air encephalography. However, the growth of this technique has taken place without full appreciation of the relatively high levels of patient dose involved. A recent national survey of CT practice in the UK has indicated that such procedures now represent about 2% of the annual total of all x-ray examinations, yet account for approximately 20% of the resulting collective dose.[9] The typical levels of patient dose from CT are relatively large compared with those for many conventional x-ray examinations of similar regions of the body, a factor which must be taken into account alongside the greater clinical value. (Table 5.2).

Such a superficial comparison of imaging modalities ignores the superior clinical information available from CT, although it serves to illustrate that doses from modern computer-based techniques of radiography are not inherently low. CT is therefore worthy of particular attention in terms of radiation protection, to ensure proper control of all exposures to patients, as well as ensuring the protection of staff and the environment. However, a CT examination does allow a reduction in dose when compared with lateral pelvimetry for pelvic outlet measurements.

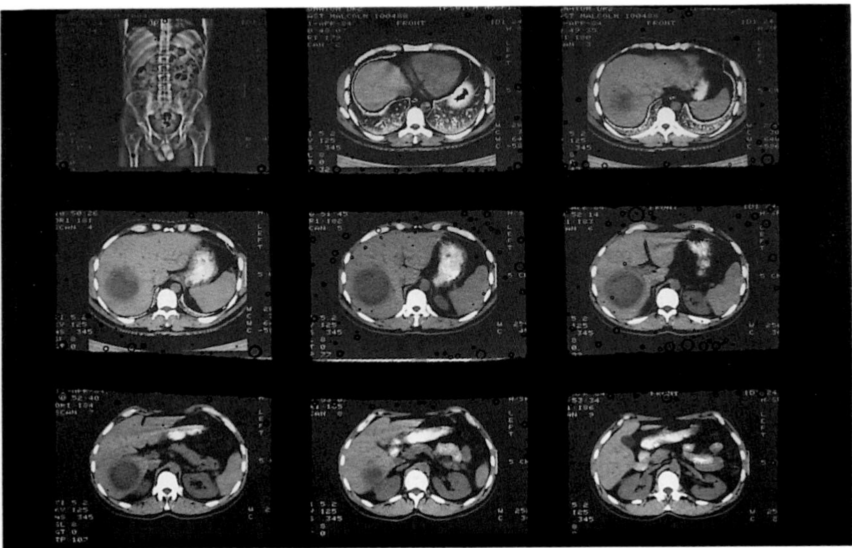

Computed tomography showing dark circular lesion within the liver (on the left of these pictures) due to an amoebic cyst

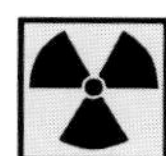

Table 5.2
Comparison between typical levels of patient dose from rotational CT[10] and conventional x-ray (Conv)[11] procedures in the UK

Examination	*Effective dose equivalent (mSv)*	
	CT[(a)]	*Conv[(b)]*
Head	3.5	0.2
Cervical spine	1.9	-
Thoracic spine	7.8	0.9
Chest	9.1	0.05
Abdomen	8.8	1.4
Lumbar spine	6.0	2.2
Pelvis	9.4	1.2
Intravenous urography	-	4.4
Barium meal	-	3.8
Barium enema	-	7.7
Cholangiography/ cholecystography	-	1.2

Notes:

(a) Representative data for complete rotational CT series in the UK taking into account the variations in both dose and utilisation between scanners in CT survey.

(b) Average data complete examinations from a previous national patient dose survey.

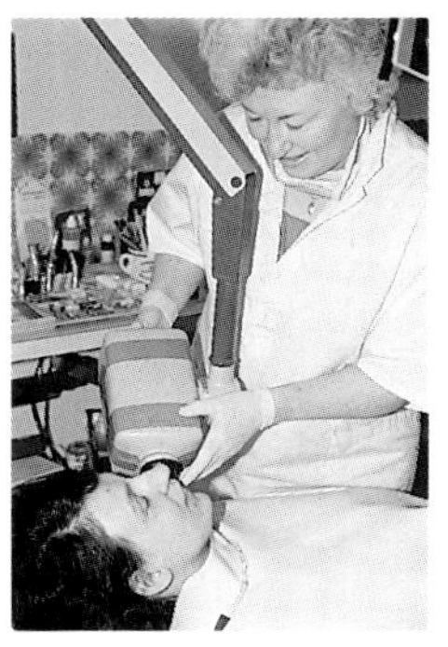

Dental x-rays account for 1% of the annual collective dose from medical x-ray examinations in the UK

A joint report from the Royal College of Radiologists and National Radiological Protection Board (NRPB) recommended that because of the potential implications of high doses in CT examinations, all patients should be individually selected for CT by experienced radiologists.[12] The suggestion has also been made that about two-thirds of the workload of a scanner at an average District General Hospital would be better undertaken, when clinically appropriate by magnetic resonance imaging (MRI), or alternative techniques not involving ionising radiation, with considerable savings in collective dose.[13] Current UK legislation[14,15] already requires that diagnostic x-ray equipment should be designed, constructed, installed, maintained and used so that all examinations are carried out with the minimum amount of radiation necessary. Comprehensive quality assurance programmes should be performed for all scanners in clinical use, covering all aspects of operation, including regular quality control measurements of imaging performance according to the recommendations of manufacturers and the Institute of Physical Sciences in Medicine.[16] All staff directing CT examinations should have received adequate special training. Effective quality assurance also requires determined managerial effort and should be a multidisciplinary activity involving all staff associated with providing the service. The final responsibility, however, rests with the radiologist who is the clinical head of department.[17]

Therapeutic x-ray machines

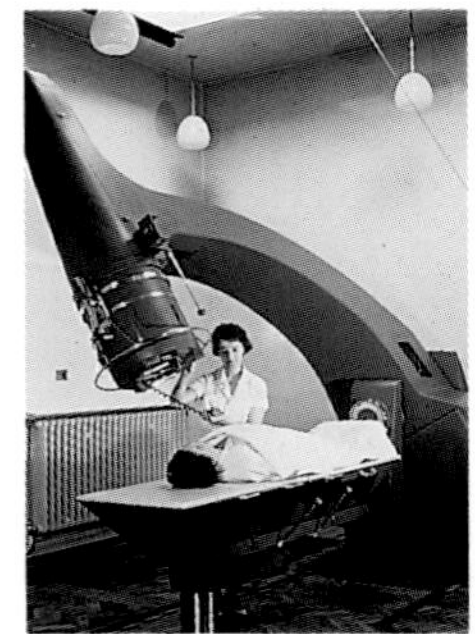

Radiotherapy: therapeutic x-ray machines are used to treat cancer

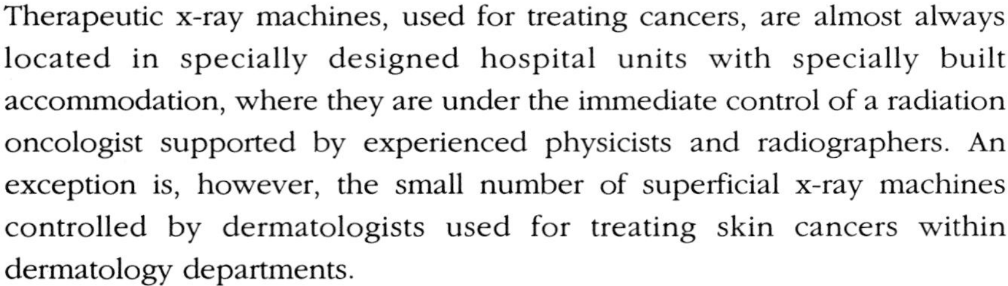

Therapeutic x-ray machines, used for treating cancers, are almost always located in specially designed hospital units with specially built accommodation, where they are under the immediate control of a radiation oncologist supported by experienced physicists and radiographers. An exception is, however, the small number of superficial x-ray machines controlled by dermatologists used for treating skin cancers within dermatology departments.

Radiotherapy machines work at somewhat higher energies than diagnostic x-ray machines, usually of the order of from 3keV to several mega electron volts (1MeV = 1000keV) and may produce electromagnetic radiation (ie x-rays) or accelerated particles such as electrons. The absorbed dose in the target tissue is necessarily large, however some healthy tissues are invariably irradiated, and there is a small risk of inducing cancer in them.

Radiotherapy departments operate with strict controls and working patterns which prevent unauthorised access to treatment rooms, and limit the potential exposure of staff. Equipment rooms are constructed to prevent or reduce to a minimum unwanted exposure, often with concrete walls several feet thick. Design must take into account not only immediate staff in the department, but others such as gardeners who may work immediately outside the treatment rooms.

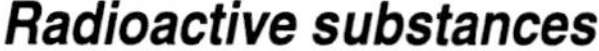

Radioactive substances

Sealed sources

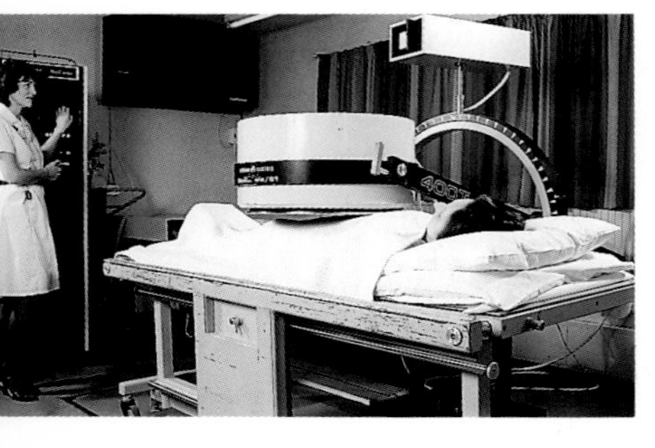

Unsealed radioactive materials are used in diagnosis. The distribution of the radioactive material is detected by a gamma camera

Sealed sources are radioactive substances enclosed in impervious, unbreakable cases. Teletherapy apparatus uses sources such as cobalt or caesium, which have long half lives of several years, and may emit radiations of high energies. Usually the sources used emit electromagnetic radiation and particles of a similar type and energy to those from x-ray machines. Each apparatus is subject to the same safety controls as radiotherapy x-ray machines.

Brachytherapy sources are used close to the tissues to be irradiated; either applied to the surface of the body or introduced into tissues or a body cavity. These sources are physically small and those with a long half life, such as cobalt, caesium or tantalum are removed from the body after the necessary dose has been given. Others, such as gold or californium, have much shorter half lives, usually a few days and quickly become relatively inert in terms of radioactive emission. They can therefore safely remain in the tissues indefinitely rather than having to be removed, provided their casing does not provoke a tissue reaction.

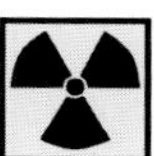

Unsealed sources

Unsealed radioactive sources may be incorporated into the body by a number of routes including ingestion, inhalation, injection into the blood, or directly into body cavities. Their use in diagnosis and therapy depends on the fact that chemically they are indistinguishable from the same substance in a non-radioactive form. In 1992 imaging procedures accounted for 89% of the work, 8% were for non-imaging diagnostic procedures and 3% for therapeutic applications.[18] An example of therapeutic application is in the treatment of thyrotoxicosis, or well differentiated thyroid tumours, using radioactive iodine which is concentrated within the thyroid gland delivering radiation locally. In therapeutic applications large doses of radioactive substances may be used.

Table 5.3
Procedure and collective doses for some of the most frequently performed nuclear medicine diagnostic procedures in 1990

Procedure	*Radionuclide*	*Radio-pharmaceutical*	*Procedure Dose (mSv)*	*Collective Dose (man Sv)*
Bone scan	^{99m}Tc	Phosphate	4.4	620.0
Lung perfusion scan	^{99m}Tc	MAA	1.0	51.0
Kidney scan	^{99m}Tc	DTPA	1.2	24.0
Thyroid scan	^{99m}Tc	Pertechnetate	1.1	21.0
Lung ventilation scan	^{81m}Kr	Gas	0.13	2.1
Kidney scan	^{99m}Tc	DMSA	1.3	19.0

Key:
^{99m}Tc - Technetium-99m: ^{81m}Kr - Krypton-81m: MAA - macroaggregated albumin:
DTPA - diethylenetriaminepentaacetic acid: DMSA - dimercaptosuccinic acid
Source: JS Hughes and M C O 'Riodan, Radiation Exposure of the UK Population - 1993 Review.

Unsealed radioactive sources are used much more widely in diagnosis, but in much smaller doses[19] (Table 5.3). The distribution of the radioactive substances in the body is identical to that of the non-radioactive counterpart, so providing a non-invasive, dynamic way of assessing the distribution of the normal substance. Such radiopharmaceuticals are now widely used in many diagnostic procedures, including bone and liver scans for detecting abnormal areas of tissue in the diagnosis of cancer. Their preparation is normally carried out in an appropriately designed laboratory, and they are administered most frequently in nuclear medicine departments, or radiology departments, although occasionally they may be administered in wards. After the radioisotope has been allowed to distribute within the patient, usually after a few hours, the patient is examined with a detector such as a gamma camera, which locates the radioactive source. Alternatively, physiological specimens may be collected, such as blood or urine, and analysed in the laboratory. Throughout the process the patient and the samples will be radioactive. Although most isotopes used in this way have a short half-life, some radioactivity remains after the investigation is completed. This may be when the patient returns to his ward or returns home, possibly using public transport, and so may expose other patients or members of the public to radiation. Appropriate provisions are made to control such unwanted exposure.[20]

Apart from the radioactive material in patients, other risks of nuclear medicine arise from contamination of work surfaces in pharmacies and laboratories and other areas, owing to spills of radioactive material. Laboratories and other working areas used for the manipulation of unsealed sources should have smooth and non-absorbent surfaces for the room, benches, tables and seats, so that they can be cleaned and decontaminated easily. Members of staff should wear protective clothing and waterproof gloves. All manipulations should be carried out over a drip tray lined with absorbent paper in order to minimise the spread of contamination due to breakages or spills.[21] Expert advice is available from the NHS Estates Management on the structure of laboratories and pharmacies and also about the amount of radioactive material which can be discharged to the drainage system or through fume cupboards into the atmosphere.[22,23] Departments handling radioactive material have to store any surplus until it has decayed to an acceptably safe level.

Sources of medical non-ionising radiation

As well as radiation from x-ray equipment and radioactive sources hospitals and clinics may include a number of other sources of radiation. Ultrasound equipment uses high frequency sound, while magnetic resonance imaging uses strong magnetic fields and radio frequency pulses.

Ultrasound

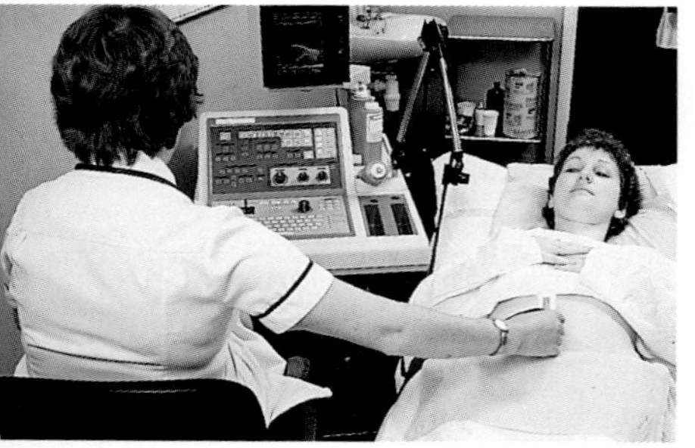

Some concern has arisen recently that the frequent use of ultrasound imaging in pregancy may have an adverse effect on foetal growth

Ultrasound imaging is widely used in clinical practice and may replace ionising radiation methods in some circumstances. This technique is particularly valuable as a diagnostic tool in obstetrics. With the information it provides, any appropriate action can be taken to improve the outcome of pregnancy. Some concern has arisen recently, however, that the frequent and repeated use of ultrasound imaging in pregnancy may have an adverse effect of foetal growth. Further studies are required to confirm these findings, however, in the meantime it would seem prudent to keep ultrasound examinations of the foetus to a minimum.[24]

Electromagnetic fields

When a biological organism is exposed to an electromagnetic field, an internal field is included within the object. The magnitude and the distribution of the internal electromagnetic energy depends on the relation between the magnitude, frequency and direction of the external field and

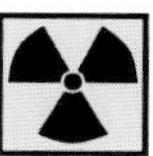

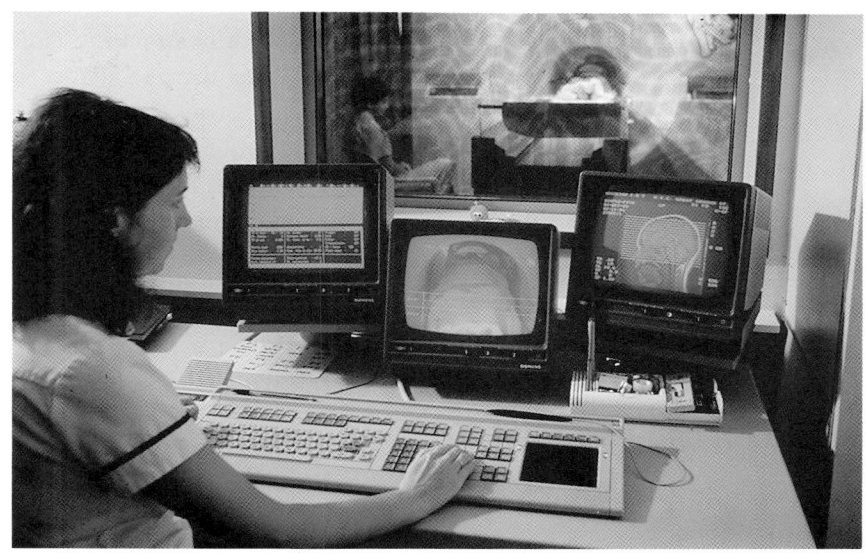

Magnetic resonance imaging equipment

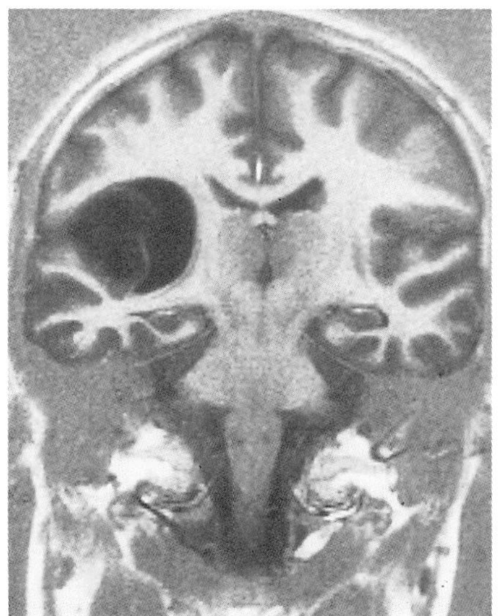

Magnetic resonance coronal scan showing large glioma (dark area on the left of the picture)

the size, shape, and anatomy of the body. Depending on the dielectric properties of the tissues, internal field energy is converted into thermal energy resulting in a local or systemic rise in temperature.[25] Although occupational exposure limits should be well below exposure levels, they may be able to induce a general rise in temperature.

High frequency electromagnetic fields (frequency range 300kHz and 300MHz) are used in physiotherapy. Concern has been expressed over the exposure of physiotherapists to high-frequency electromagnetic fields during diathermic treatment. Studies carried out in Denmark to assess the possible relationship between such exposure and congenital malformations have so far been inconclusive.[26]

The strong magnetic field generated by magnetic resonance (MR) imaging is generally considered to be safe both for patients undergoing MR examination and for health practitioners using the technique. A study of the safety considerations in MR imaging[27] concluded that in some areas the potentially harmful effects of MR imaging are not yet definitively known. Studies into the effects of MR imaging are continuing and in addition a large case-control study of childhood cancer and magnetic fields associated with electricity transmission is currently in progress. The possibility that exposure to electromagnetic fields generated by powerlines and domestic wiring causes cancers, including childhood cancer, is one of continuing public concern and scientific debate.[28]

Lasers too use electromagnetic non-ionising radiation. These however, are recognised as being able to damage tissue, and are often used in medicine specifically to remove tissue. The use of lasers in medical practice is well controlled in order to avoid hazards to patients and staff from the risk of injury, in particular to the eye, which can result from lack of protective measures, the use of faulty laser equipment, misdirected beams or inappropriate laser control settings. Guidance on the safe use of lasers in medical practice has been published by the Department of Health.[29] The British Standards Institute also publishes standards on the safe use of lasers.

Sources of non-medical ionising radiation

In this chapter we have only considered in detail the population's exposure to ionising radiation through health care. It should be remembered that the total amount of exposure for an individual will include a number of other sources such as natural radioactivity within the human body itself, building materials, radioactive substances used by nuclear industry, nuclear power generation, and even nuclear warfare.

Who is at risk?

In 1990 a report of the joint working party between the Royal College of Radiologists and the NRPB was published and concluded that it would not be unreasonable to suggest that at least 20% of x-ray examinations carried out in the UK are clinically unhelpful, because they are unlikely to give information which would be useful for patient management.[30] Any unnecessary exposure to ionising radiation places both patients and staff at risk. This is contrary to the requirements of the Ionising Radiation Regulations (1988) and the recommendations of the International Commission on Radiological Protection in respect of dose limitation. In response to these findings the joint working party recommended rapid dissemination of the Royal College of Radiologists booklet containing guidelines for 12 types of radiographic examination.[31] The guidelines aim to encourage more appropriate use of diagnostic radiology and so reduce the performance of unnecessary x-ray examinations. Since publication of the guidelines the working party of the Royal College of Radiologists and others have found dramatic reductions in referral rates following compliance with the guidelines. However, the introduction of guidelines on its own may only have a transient effect without effective monitoring of practice and peer review. Without such assurance of compliance with an agreed standard of practice, good practice is unlikely to be translated into common practice.[32]

The most likely reason for patients, staff or the public being unintentionally exposed to radiation is probably human error. (see box on page 67).

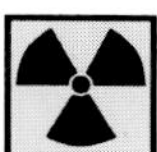

Possible causes of unnecessary or unintentional exposure to radiation in health care

- Unnecessary investigation
- Design failure
- Faulty construction or positioning of equipment
- Inadequate protection arrangements
- Miscalculation of radiation dose or exposure limits
- Loss of patients' records leading to repeat investigations

Unnecessary or unintentional exposure to ionising radiation

The public, patients and health care staff are potentially at risk from the environmental effects of the use of radiation in health care.

Patients

The use of ionising radiation for diagnostic or therapeutic purposes is intended to benefit the patient and the doses given are controlled by the 1985 and 1988 Ionising Radiation Regulations, and the Administration of Radioactive Substances Regulations (1978), all of which include the principle of ALARA (as low as reasonably achievable).[33,34] Outdated treatments have been followed by the development of secondary cancers: ie, the irradiation of 'enlarged thymus' in small infants, treatment of scalp ringworm by superficial x-rays, and over-use of diagnostic x-rays when, for example, following up patients with pulmonary tuberculosis, or using barium studies to investigate gastro-intestinal problems. Fortunately, treatment of thyrotoxicosis with radioiodine has not to date been shown to cause leukaemia or thyroid cancer.

A patient may be inappropriately exposed in an x-ray or nuclear medicine department or ward as a result of inadequate protection or unsatisfactory schemes of work. In most such instances the dose received is a very small proportion of the dose that should have been received by the patient for his or her own potential benefit. However, the dose needed in a therapeutic procedure is some 1000-fold greater than in a diagnostic procedure and most patients who are seriously over exposed have been receiving radiotherapy. One such example in Exeter, arose from arithmetical errors in the calibration of radiotherapy equipment, which was not checked by an independent person or confirmed by physical measurement in the department.[35] The error was not recognised for many years, during which time many patients were treated.

In nuclear medicine practice, patients may be exposed to radiation from isotopes in other patients. An example of this risk might arise when a patient has been given a therapy dose of an unsealed radionuclide eg ^{131}I. Such patients should be given a single room with its own toilet and washing facilities. The room should incorporate adequate radiation shielding and nursing procedures must take account of the risk to staff.[36]

Health care staff

Doses received by radiation workers within the NHS have been recorded for many years. About 99% of all medical workers receive annual doses below 1mSv and only 0.1% receive more than 5 mSv. A survey by the National Radiological Protection Board showed that occupational doses received by workers in the nuclear industry have continued to decline steadily and are now about half of the values recorded in 1987.[37] This has been largely due to dose management programmes that have led to improved practice. Even so the doses were appreciably larger than those received by NHS staff.

Members of staff in hospitals and clinics, or in general medical and dental practice are potentially at risk of exposure to ionising radiation, although most workers receive little or no occupational exposure. The risk is likely

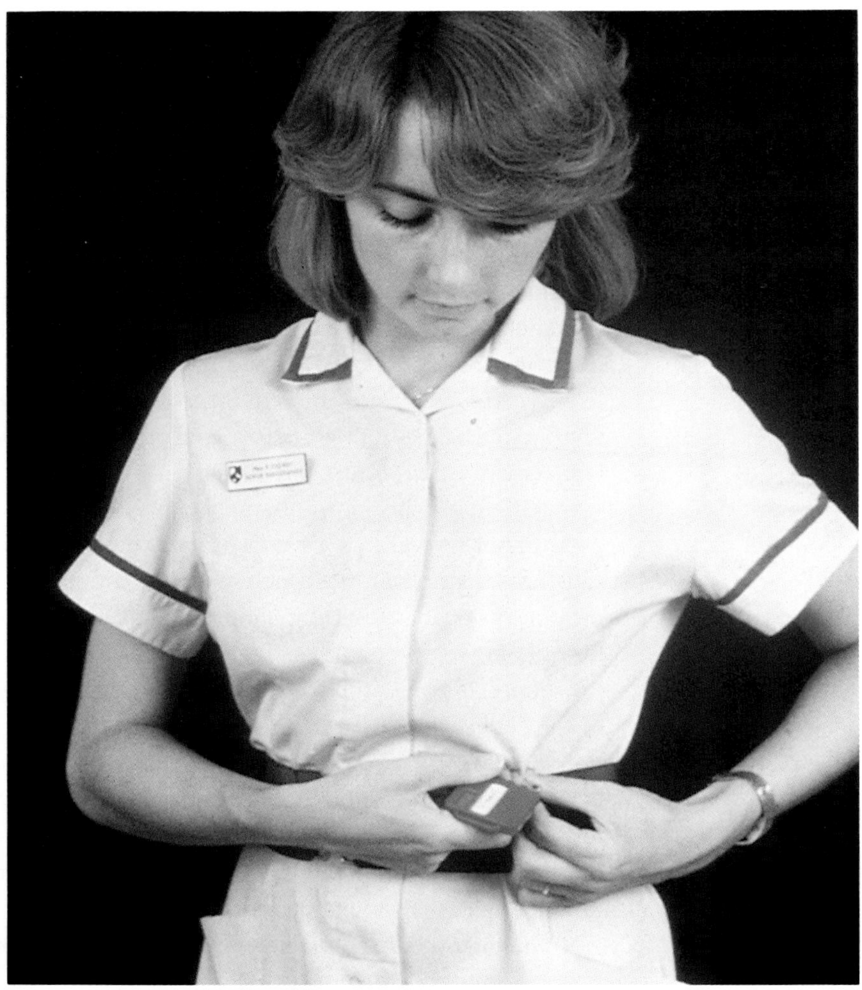

Radiation badges are worn by staff to help monitor their levels of radiation exposure

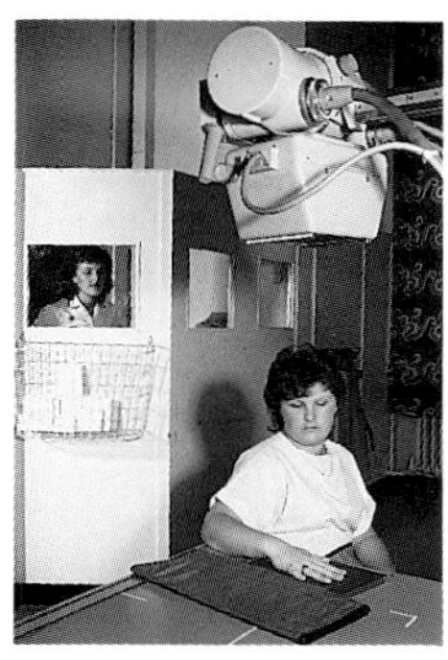

Health care staff should be protected from radiation by standing behind lead shields or wearing lead aprons when operating equipment

to be low for those who only use public areas; somewhat greater in those working in wards or operating theatres, where mobile x-ray machines and/or radioactive substances are in use; and of significantly greater for workers in x-ray or nuclear medicine departments. Personal dosimetry is a useful check on working procedures and provides reassurance for members of staff. The close monitoring of exposure over many years has shown that the risk of significant exposure is very small unless there has been inadequate protection, poor instruction and/or inadequate schemes of work.

The public

Members of the public entering hospital premises may be exposed to ionising radiations in the event of a failure of any of the safety arrangements previously described. Visitors to hospitals may be exposed by being close to patients who are undergoing nuclear medical investigations or systemic, interstitial or intracavitary radiotherapy. This problem can be alleviated with appropriate advice to relatives about the length of time of visits and the distance that the visitor should keep from the patient. Provided that advice is observed, the dose received by visitors will be less than the permissible dose prescribed in the Ionising Radiation Regulations (1988), so it is unlikely to have any untoward consequences. With the rare exception of patients who have undergone neutron activation analysis as a diagnostic procedure, and who may therefore be radioactive, only those patients who have had radionuclides incorporated physiologically or inserted into their body cavities are likely to be radioactive. Relatives of such patients who are at risk are, firstly, very young children (who should not normally be breast fed or come into close contact with the radioactive parent) and, secondly, others in the immediate family.[38] Very ill patients whose relatives have been appropriately counselled about the small risk should be allowed 'close' visiting. Such visitors may be exposed to some radiation, but this is unlikely to have any serious after-effects, and in such circumstances they may wish to accept the risk.

Control of exposure to ionising radiation

Regulations

Several sources of advice are available about the risks of exposure to ionising radiation, notably the International Commission on Radiological Protection (ICRP). This body regularly receives reports on the effects of exposure to ionising radiation and gives advice about the risks. In the United Kingdom the National Radiological Protection Board interprets the reports and advice of the ICRP and similar bodies and in turn advises government departments, in particular, the Department of Health and the Health and Safety Commission of the Department of Trade and Industry, about the rules and regulations required for the safety of the population as a whole and individual sectors of the population.

The Ionising Radiation Regulations (1985), and the Ionising Radiation (Protection of Persons Undergoing Medical Examination or Treatment) Regulations (1988) are framed to create safe practices in order that ionising radiation doses to patients are kept to a minimum and that workers and the general public are not exposed to doses likely to lead to any significant harm to their health. Following these regulations, associated guidelines, such as the Health and Safety Commission's *Approved Code of Practice*[39] were produced to clarify and make practical the regulations. The keeping, disposal and use of radioactive material is regulated by the Radioactive Substance Act (1960), revised in 1991. Transfer and transport of radioactive materials is also covered by a number of statutory instruments.[40] Administration of radioactive materials to patients and research subjects is regulated by the Medicines (Administration of Radioactive Substances) Regulations (1978).

Background to radiation protection

The data informing these regulations and guidelines is derived from a number of sources. The main source of information on risk of radiation-induced cancer following exposure to whole-body gamma radiation comes from follow-up studies on the survivors of the atomic bombs at Hiroshima and Nagasaki. Information on the effects of incorporated alpha emitters comes from miners exposed to radon and its decay products, from workers exposed to radium in the luminising industry, from patients given radium-224 for treatment of disease and from patients given the x-ray contrast medium thorotrast. Information on risk is reviewed periodically by the United Nations Scientific Committee on the Effects of Atomic Radiation (UNSCEAR) which publishes its reports to the General Assembly.

Assessments of cancer risks derived from the Japanese populations and other groups are based mostly on exposures at high doses delivered over a short period of time. In practice, most people are exposed to low levels of radiation over long periods of time. It is generally assumed that there is a simple proportional relationship between dose and risk, and that there is no threshold below which cancers and hereditary effects do not occur,[41] although somatic effects such as cataracts, and skin erythema do have a dose limit, below which they are unlikely to occur.

Radiological protection is based on three central requirements (see box on page 71). The first requirement emphasises the obvious need to consider harmful effects before deciding whether to use a procedure involving exposure to ionising radiation. Since it is assumed that no radiation dose is entirely free from risk, it is not enough merely to comply with a limit. Doses below the limit also need consideration and should be reduced whenever and wherever they can. However, the point must come where further reductions would be unreasonable in terms of social and economic cost. The third requirement of radiological protection is concerned with not

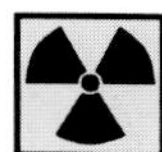

Principle requirements of radiological protection as expressed by the International Commission on Radiological Protection

- No practice shall be adopted unless its introduction produces a positive net benefit.
- All exposures shall be kept as low as reasonably achievable, economic and social factors being taken into account.
- The dose equivalent to individuals shall not exceed the limits recommended for the appropriate circumstances by the Commission.

exposing any individuals and their descendants to what is considered to be an unacceptable degree of risk. Strict limits are imposed which specify the effective dose equivalent that a person may receive. For occupationally exposed persons the NRPB recommends an annual dose limit of 20mSv. For female workers, the ICRP recommends that once pregnancy has been confirmed, the dose limit of 2mSv to the surface of the woman's abdomen should apply for the remainder of the pregnancy. The NRPB however, believe that the principle of ALARA should be applied. It would then be unlikely that exposures would be above 1mSv. For members of the public the ICRP and the NRPB recommend an overall limit of 1mSv per year.[42] For exposures of patients during medical use of radiation, however, dose limits do not apply.[43] The elements of control in this case are the justification for the exposure and minimisation of doses and risks. Patients should not be exposed to doses higher than those required for effective diagnosis or treatment. Since total protection is not possible, again the principle of ALARA has to be applied.[44]

The above constraints presume that any exposure of a patient, for medical reasons, is for his or her either potential or definite benefit. In addition, the National Radiological Protection Board and Royal College of Radiologists have published advice on the use of ionising radiation, particularly in diagnostic procedures, emphasising the practices likely to minimise exposures. Any circumstances in which a person receives an inappropriate amount of radiation, or where the dose to a patient is in excess of, or significantly less than, that which was intended, should be investigated. The reason for the wrong dose may be a design fault or failure, such as a miscalculation of the amount of shielding material required; damaged, wrongly positioned or deteriorated protective material; failure to close a protective door; or deterioration of a protective apron.

Safe systems of work

In many circumstances radiological protection depends on well established work schemes and inappropriate exposure often arises because these are not properly followed. Such schemes are based on physical principles, and are to be followed in detail both in normal working practice and abnormal eventualities. Sealed sources may leak radiation when their protective covering has been breached in any way, large sources may become stuck in transit between their safe and active positions, small sources may be lost, for example, by being discarded inadvertently in dressings. All patients who have undergone systemic treatment with radioactive substances, and those who have had diagnostic investigations from radioisotopes, will remain radioactive for some time — the latter for a shorter time. Their body waste might also be radioactive. The bodies of deceased patients may be a potential source of danger to physicians, embalmers and crematoria attendants. The Ionising Radiation Regulations (1985) define the time which must pass after the injection of radioactive substances, and the maximum activity permissible before embalming or cremation. Appropriate schemes of work can take account of all these potential sources of hazard and therefore allow risks to be controlled.

Discussion

The physical properties of ionising radiations, in particular their ability to penetrate materials and their rate of radioactive decay, make it impossible to guarantee that their medical use will have no consequences for the environment. In most cases the doses involved are very small — less than those contributed by natural background radiation. As the risks of detectable changes from exposure to ionising radiation are approximately proportional to the dose received, the biological effects are also in consequence likely to be very small indeed.

For patients who are undergoing diagnosis or treatment with ionising radiation, it is normally accepted that the danger to them is outweighed by the potential or actual benefits of the procedure. Every effort is made to keep the doses employed as low as possible without detriment to the medical effect required. Doctors who use ionising radiations in the investigation or treatment of patients are expected to consider other methods not requiring ionising radiation such as ultrasound, magnetic resonance imaging, endoscopy, or surgical procedures although they may have their own inherent risks. Persons other than patients under-going treatment should be protected by the methods described earlier, including the use of shielding, by being kept at a safe distance, and by appropriate training, safe schemes of work for staff and monitoring of exposure levels. Outdated equipment should also be replaced. The inevitable cost of safety measures to reduce further the risks to patients, staff, the public and the environment, should not be used to justify inaction.

CHAPTER 6

Microbial hazards

Development, spread and control of infection

Clinical areas

Infection can be spread in hospital environments by airborne micro-organisms, by direct contact between patients and staff, and by indirect contact — via the surfaces of contaminated instruments for example. Patients, staff, medical instruments, and the hospital building itself can all act as reservoirs for micro-organisms and as potential sources of infection. Hospital acquired infections in patients are usually a consequence of serious illness, surgery or treatment that reduce a person's immune defences. Such infections are often caused by normal commensal organisms. Although healthy staff and visitors to a hospital face a much lower risk of infection than such patients, health care workers are exposed to some risks not usually encountered by patients, for example through repeated exposures to body fluids that may be infected.

Control of infection in hospitals is the responsibility of local committees set up as the result of a recommendation of the Control Health Services Council in 1959 (see box on page 74). The efficacy of such infection surveillance and control programmes has been established through the measurement of the inverse relation between their implementation in a hospital and the incidence of hospital acquired infections in that hospital.[1]

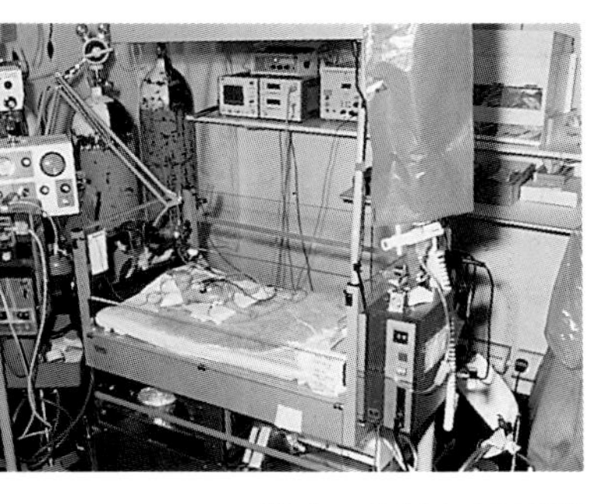

Newborn babies, especially those in intensive care, are particularly vulnerable to infection

Although only hospitals and other provider units providing acute services are required to have an infection control team (ie a consultant with responsibility for infection control and one or more infection control nurses), small and long stay hospitals should make formal arrangements to receive infection control advice, both routinely and in an outbreak, from a local infection control team.

Infection control in hospitals

- Control of infection committees are responsible for infection control in hospitals
- These committees are chaired by a control of infection officer, who may be a medical microbiologist
- They are responsible for the protection of staff and patients, education of staff, and surveillance of procedures, including the production of an outbreak plan
- Infection control nurses carry out many of the day to day functions
- Occupational health physicians have a complementary function in the immunisation and surveillance of staff
- The consultant in communicable disease control (CCDC) must be a member of the hospital infection control committee in order that they may make a judgement on any implications for the community of an outbreak of infection and act accordingly.

Non-clinical areas

Outside the clinical areas of hospitals, laboratory staff and others face a risk of infection. Microbiologists will have to isolate and culture human pathogens and laboratory staff handle blood and other potentially infective fluids. Pathogenic agents can be inhaled from infected aerosols and splashes generated when liquids are processed, or when spillages occur. The skin of staff working in laboratories may become contaminated, with abrasions providing a means of entry to the body. Guidelines exist for controlling infection among laboratory workers and strict adherence to them should eliminate many of the risks.

Mortuary technicians and pathologists come into contact with infected bodies, and by the use of drills and bone-saws during postmortem examinations, particles of infected tissue can be distributed. Most organisms in cadavers are not infectious to healthy staff with intact skins, but there are specific risks in dealing with the bodies of individuals who have had communicable diseases such as, hepatitis B, tuberculosis and Creutzfeldt-Jakob disease. A report by the Health and Safety Advisory Committee gives guidance on the infection risks in post-mortem room practice.[2] The report details the identification and assessment of risk and gives standards for safe working practices. The report also highlights the importance of adequate occupational health facilities for all mortuary staff. Employers must ensure that occupational health arrangements include agreed immunisation procedures, eg against hepatitis B. Because of the risk of staff acquiring pulmonary tuberculosis by the airborne route, it is important that all mortuary staff be provided with tuberculin testing, BCG immunisation and chest x-ray where appropriate. Health Building Note 20

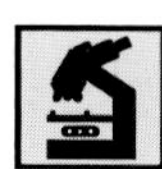

gives guidance on the design and construction of mortuaries and post-mortem rooms both in the preparation of new and upgrading of existing facilities.[3] The risks of HIV (human immunodeficiency virus) infection to mortuary technicians and pathologists have been reviewed,[4] with the conclusion that HIV postmortem work is safe when carried out in accordance with Health and Safety Advisory Committee guidance.[5]

Beyond the hospital

The risks of infection spreading outside the confines of a hospital are low (with the exception of secondary person-to-person spread). In most cases, a meaningful risk of infection in the neighbourhood of a hospital would imply an extraordinarily high risk to those working inside the building. Some cases of legionnaire's disease have been attributed to contaminated hospital cooling towers but overall the risks are no greater than those associated with any other large public building or certain industrial processes. The consultant in communicable disease control, who is a member of the hospital infection control committee, has responsibility for any outbreak of infection or incident within a hospital that has implications for the community.

There are, however, circumstances in which infected materials may move from the hospital into the community. Acute care hospitals generate 5-6 kg of solid waste per patient everyday, but the bulk of it does not pose any greater risk of infection than does general domestic waste. If staff carry out control procedures and known infected material is contained until it is decontaminated, there should be no general risk to the public. Laboratory samples are sometimes transported as pathological specimens by post, and require special packaging to prevent any leakage and risk of infection. Soiled and fouled laundry is potentially infectious, especially if it has been used by patients with communicable diseases. The contracting out of hospital laundry services creates a potential risk of spreading infection into the community, but only if the laundry does not follow appropriate infection control procedures.

Airborne infection

Tuberculosis

Tuberculosis was a very common problem in the past and probably still presents the major risk of airborne infection among hospital staff. Fortunately, its prevalence among hospital staff has fallen markedly in recent decades in line with the incidence in the community. This decline now appears to be slowing, however, and with the emergence of multiple drug resistant organisms, tuberculosis could once more become a major public health hazard. Indeed, the incidence of tuberculosis among some inner city communities, particularly in the United States is causing concern.

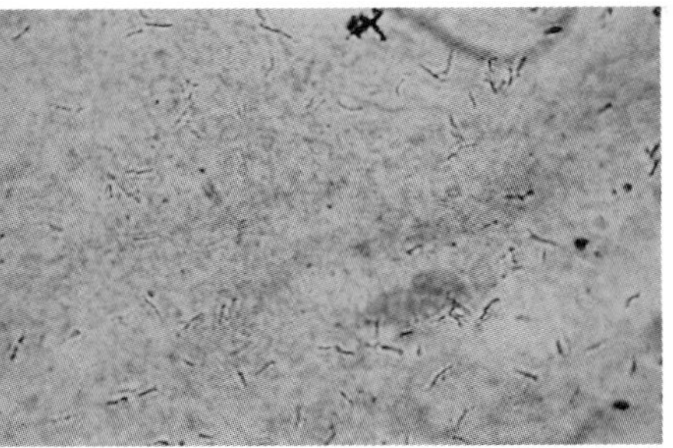

Mycobacterium tuberculosis

The major threat to health care staff comes from mycobacteria which have developed multiple resistance to drugs. This resistance to conventional drug therapy means that mycobacterial loads and infectivity remain high for a long time. Multiple drug resistant mycobacteria are usually isolated from immunocompromised patients with other illnesses who require intensive nursing and medical support, and hence close contact between staff and patients. Outbreaks due to multiple drug resistant strains have been reported in hospitals and prisons in other countries.[6-8] These outbreaks have affected patients with immunosuppression due to HIV infection and also health care workers. Mortality in these outbreaks has been high, and measures to control tuberculosis are being reviewed in the United States. Poor design of the ventilation systems may contribute to spread of the disease.[9] Although notification of a small number of multiple drug resistant strains have been received by the UK Mycobacterium Reference Unit from various parts of England and Wales, none has been formally reported in association with HIV infection and no outbreaks are known to have occurred.[10] However, the experience in the United States makes it essential that vigilance for such cases should be maintained and procedures to control infection reviewed.[11] Case finding should be balanced against the strategy recommended by the World Health Organisation of appropriate treatment of known cases of tuberculosis and rigorous record keeping.

Mortuary technicians and staff on infectious disease or respiratory wards are likely to be at particular risk from tuberculosis. The relative rarity of the disease now means that the diagnosis may be delayed while investigations are being carried out and this increases the time during which spread of infection can occur. Staff involved in doing bronchoscopies might be particularly liable to infection if the procedure generates aerosols containing mycobacteria. Vaccination of hospital staff and others at risk of being exposed to tuberculosis is therefore likely to become increasingly important.

Risks of health care

Microbial hazards can be associated with changes or advances in health care in several ways. The introduction of an item of equipment or process might itself pose a risk, if it is liable to be easily contaminated and so spread infection, if used to investigate or treat immunocompromised patients, for example.

The widespread use of anaesthetic equipment and ventilators in the 1950s and 1960s led to some respiratory infections in patients.[12] Gram negative bacilli, particularly *Pseudomonas*, were able to multiply inside nebulisers and other parts of the breathing circuitry and infect patients on whom the apparatus was used. Resuscitation equipment, humidification tents and other items were similarly affected. The problems were largely eliminated by design changes such as the incorporation of bacterial filters and detachable circuits for equipment in contact with the patient. Hazard analysis procedures addressing microbial risks should be routinely incorporated into the design of medical equipment and the risks have been

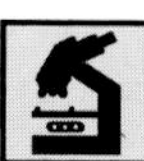

much reduced. Occasional problems with *Pseudomonas* infection still occur, however, when decontamination equipment fails, or unforseen design problems manifest themselves.[13]

The risk of nebulisers and other equipment becoming contaminated with *Legionella* has been recognised more recently. This organism multiplies in air cooling and water distribution systems and is inhaled when water from these sources forms an aerosol, for example, in showers or splashes from water taps. *Legionella* has caused infection when reusable therapeutic nebulisers were washed with contaminated tap water; these should therefore be filled and washed using only sterile fluids. Immunocompromised patients are at greatest risk, but *Legionella* can also infect healthy staff and hospital visitors. Several outbreaks of legionnaire's disease associated with hospital cooling towers and air conditioning systems.[14]

Flexible fibreoptic endoscopes are routinely used for many diagnostic and surgical procedures and pose several problems. They contain narrow channels and valves which require diligent cleaning, are fragile, cannot be heat sterilised, and are often used in a series of patients in one session. Some endoscopes require more careful decontamination than others. Colonoscopes, sigmoidoscopes and bronchoscopes require less stringent attention than arthroscopes, laparoscopes and choledochoscopes. Transmission of infection from patient-to-patient is rare if appropriate disinfection procedures are followed. Even so, cases have been reported[15] including infection with hepatitis B virus after gastrointestinal endoscopy,[16] and with *Serratia*[17,18] and *Mycobacteria*[19] after bronchoscopy. A further problem is that doctors may be confused in making a diagnosis because endoscopes become colonised with environmental organisms and as a result patient samples may be contaminated.[20] Endoscopic procedures also bring the operator into close contact with patients and potentially infectious material such as sputum, blood, and faeces.

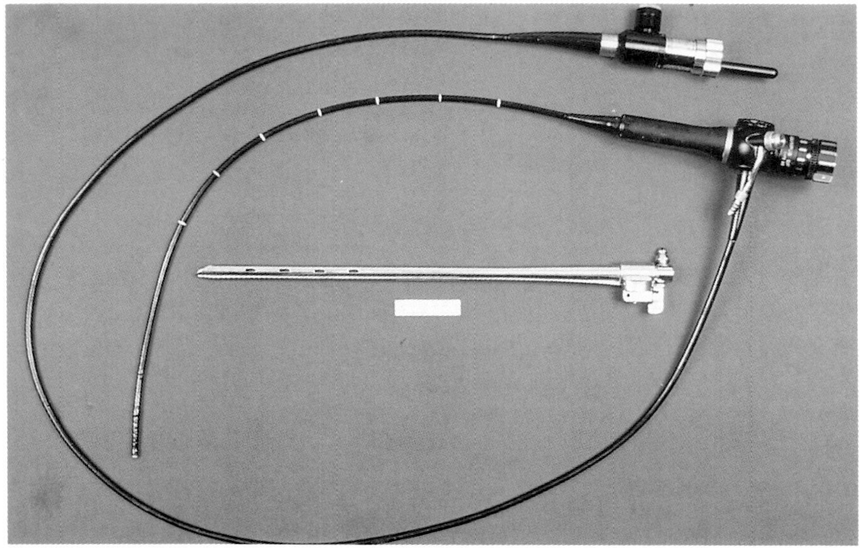

Bronchoscope

The British Society of Gastroenterology has issued guidance on the cleaning and disinfection of equipment for gastrointestinal flexible endoscopy[21] to prevent patient-to-patient and patient to staff transmission of HIV, HBV and other pathogens. The guidance recommends that all endoscopic equipment should be thoroughly mechanically cleaned with detergent and be disinfected before the endoscopy list begins, between each patient examined, and at the end of the list. The most important procedure is the mechanical cleaning of the endoscope to remove all blood, secretions and organic material, as the presence of these will prevent adequate penetration of the disinfectant, and the time required for effective disinfection may be many times that recommended for bacterial or viral inactivation.

Infection by direct contact

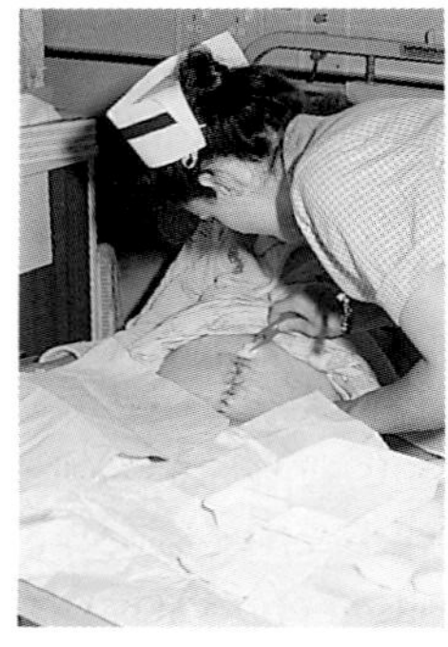

Surgical wounds may be contaminated by resident skin bacteria

The incidence of bacterial infection of surgical wounds has been reduced as a result of modern aseptic techniques, laminar flow operating theatre environments, prophylactic antibiotics, etc. Even so, some wound contamination from resident skin bacteria or from nasal commensal organisms such as *Staphylococci* is almost inevitable. The development of multiple drug resistant *Staphylococci* has caused problems in many hospitals and routine surveillance of staff is now common practice.

Bacterial septicaemia and other infections may result from the use of intravascular devices such as central venous catheters and arterial lines. Fluids for infusion can become contaminated, particularly those for total parenteral nutrition which may support the growth of micro-organisms. Bacteria can enter intravenous infusions at junctions in tubing but the site

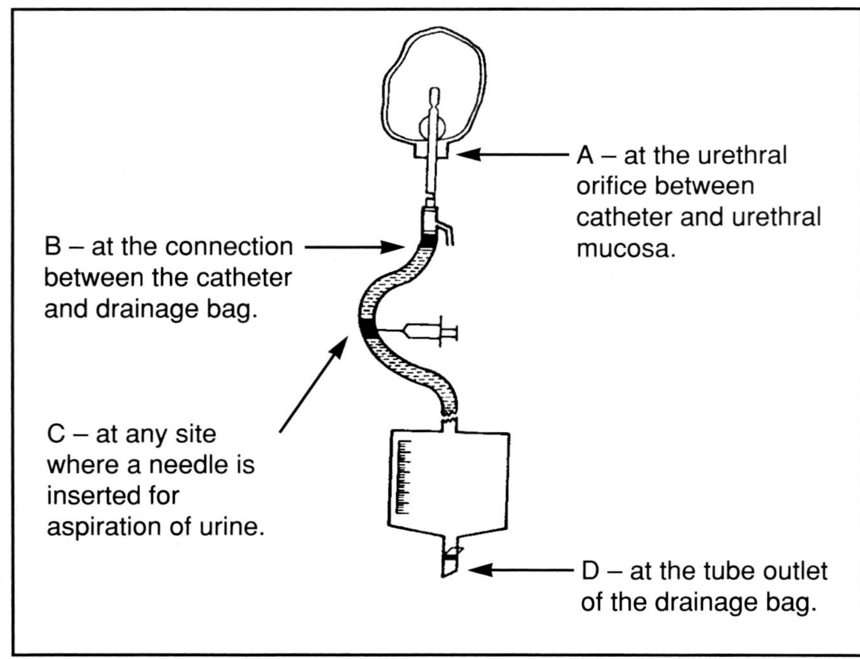

Figure 6.1: Four areas where micro-organisms can enter the urinary catheter system

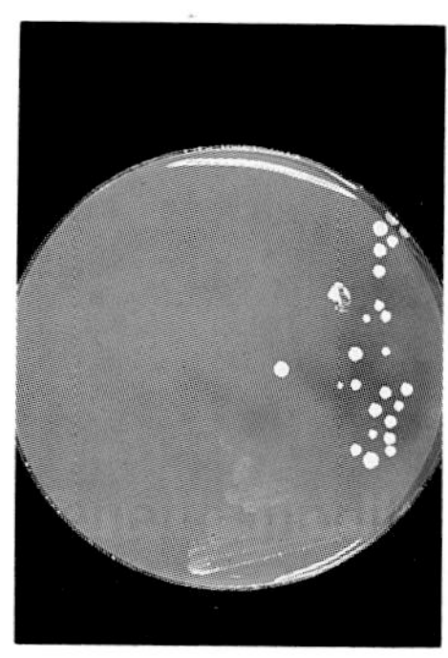

Colonies of Staphylococci *on culture plate*

of skin penetration is the most common portal of entry for organisms, or possibly from transient bacteraemia colonising the canula. Subsequent infections can occur at the entry site, in the bloodstream, or at distant sites such as heart valves.

Urinary tract infections are the most common acquired infections in hospitals, and about 90% of these are associated with urinary catheters or genitourinary surgery. Most represent endogenous infection with commensal bacteria from the gut or genito-urinary tract introduced when the catheter is inserted. Bacteria can also readily enter through the lumen of the catheter in open systems, and prolonged catheterisation means that bacterial infection is almost inevitable.

Infection from contact with blood

Contact with infected blood and blood products is recognised to be the greatest occupational hazard for health care workers. It usually occurs when the health worker's skin is broken by contact with a sharp contaminated object but can also occur when blood comes into contact with an open wound, inflamed, eczematous skin or mucous membranes, such as the eyes and mouth.

The likelihood of accidental and potentially infective contact with patient blood has increased considerably over the past 20 years. Operating sessions are longer and more complex, and many more invasive diagnostic procedures such as arteriography are being performed, as are intravascular treatments such as angioplasty. Haemodialysis and plasmapheresis require large volumes of blood to be handled and this carries a high risk.

Less dramatically, advances in diagnostic and monitoring techniques have created a demand for frequent venous blood sampling. Venepuncture carries some risk of injury and of accidental inoculation of blood and transmission of disease. This can be reduced, but not eliminated, by not resheathing needles and by careful attention to the safe use and disposal of all contaminated 'sharps'. Techniques which involve the collection of capillary blood, for example, for monitoring blood glucose, have become popular over the past decade and transmission of infection from patient-to-patient has occurred due to inappropriate reuse of a device for obtaining capillary blood.[22] More complex analytical devices for blood gas and biochemical estimations are now used outside hospital laboratories, in intensive care units and on wards, where staff are less familiar with the equipment and with correct infection control procedures than full time laboratory staff. This probably increases the risk of staff having contact with patient blood and therefore risking infection[23] and emphasises the need for adequate training in infection control procedures.

In a study in a London teaching hospital, 447 incidents of accidental contact with a patient's blood by staff were reported over a 30 month period,[24] 75% were caused by needlestick injuries or other sharp objects, and the remainder by spills, bites and scratches. Fifty five per cent occurred among nursing staff and 18% among doctors. These figures are probably

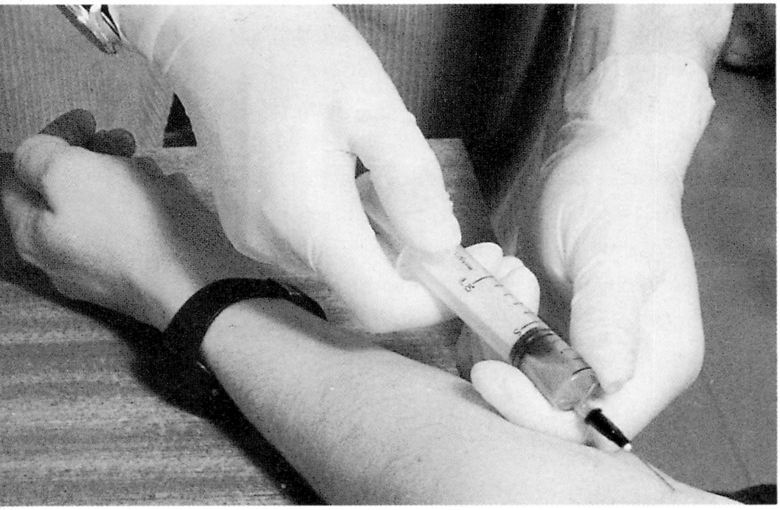

Venepuncture carries some risk of injury to health care staff including the accidental inoculation of blood and transmission of disease

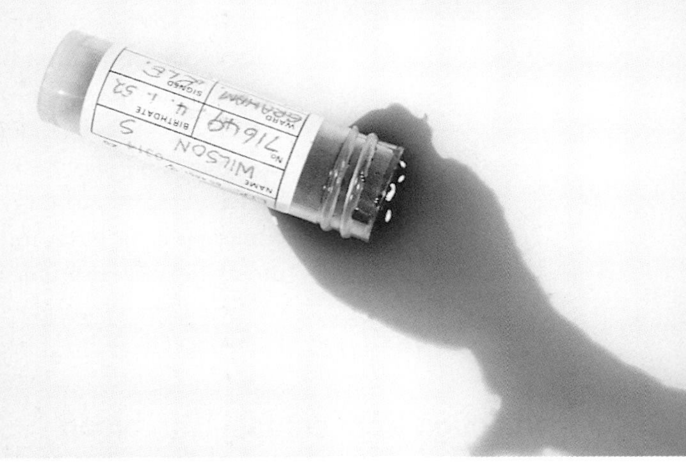

Contact with infected blood and blood products is recognised to be the greatest occupational hazard for health care workers

considerable underestimates as most incidents are not reported.[25] Often the person concerned is unaware that contact with blood has occurred.[26] A survey of sharps injuries during operations revealed that in 5.6% of operations, there was an accidental injury to either the surgeon or the assistant.[27] Surgeons' gloves have been found to be holed at the end of operating sessions, and one survey showed an overall perforation rate for all gloves as 37.5%.[28] In recent years the use of double gloving ie. wearing two pairs of gloves has been adopted by some surgical staff. In one study of double-gloving, the rate of puncture for outer gloves was lower at 11%.[29]

Viruses can be transferred when infectious blood comes into contact with the conjunctiva and mucus membranes, and there is a theoretical risk that hepatitis B and HIV may be transmitted through aerosols generated by power drills used in orthopaedic surgery and dentistry for example.[30] In practice, neither infection has been known to be transmitted in this way.

Hepatitis

The major hazard arising from contact with blood is infection with the viruses that cause hepatitis. The commonest is hepatitis B, which is present in the blood of infected patients in high concentrations for long periods in the UK; about 0.1% of the population are carriers of the virus. Hepatitis B usually causes a self limiting disease but it can occasionally be fatal or cause chronic liver disease. It is extremely infectious and possibly as little as 0.00004ml of blood is sufficient to transmit the disease from an acutely infected patient.[31] The risk of infection following exposure may reach 30%.

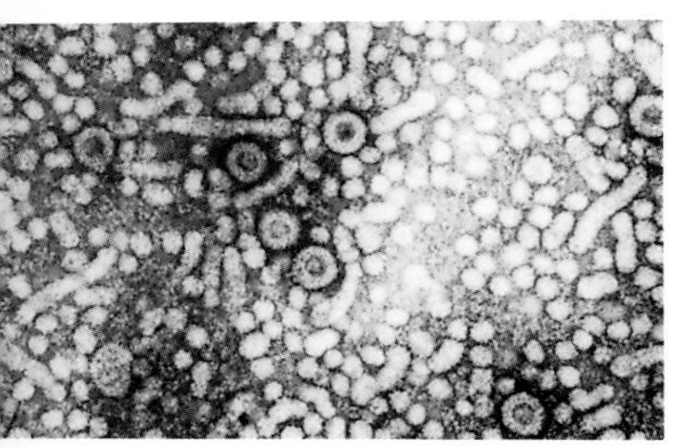

Hepatitis B virus (magnified x 66,000)

Hepatitis B occurred in almost epidemic proportions among the staff of renal units when haemodialysis was introduced in the 1960s; 122 cases and six deaths were recorded among staff in Edinburgh and Manchester.[32] The incidence of hepatitis B among health care staff has declined since then as

Clinical course of hepatitis B

Exposure

Incubation period
- infectious to others

Acute hepatitis B

66% have clinical infection
- flu-like symptoms
- 50% go on to develop jaundice

33% have subclinical infection
- asymptomatic

0.01%

Fulminant hepatitis
- usually results in death

10%

90%

Chronic carriers

50% develop chronic persistent hepatitis
- infectious to others

50% develop chronic active hepatitis
- more likely to develop serious liver damage

Recovery
- occurs within 6 months
- lifelong immunity

25%

Primary liver cancer

Cirrhosis

Death

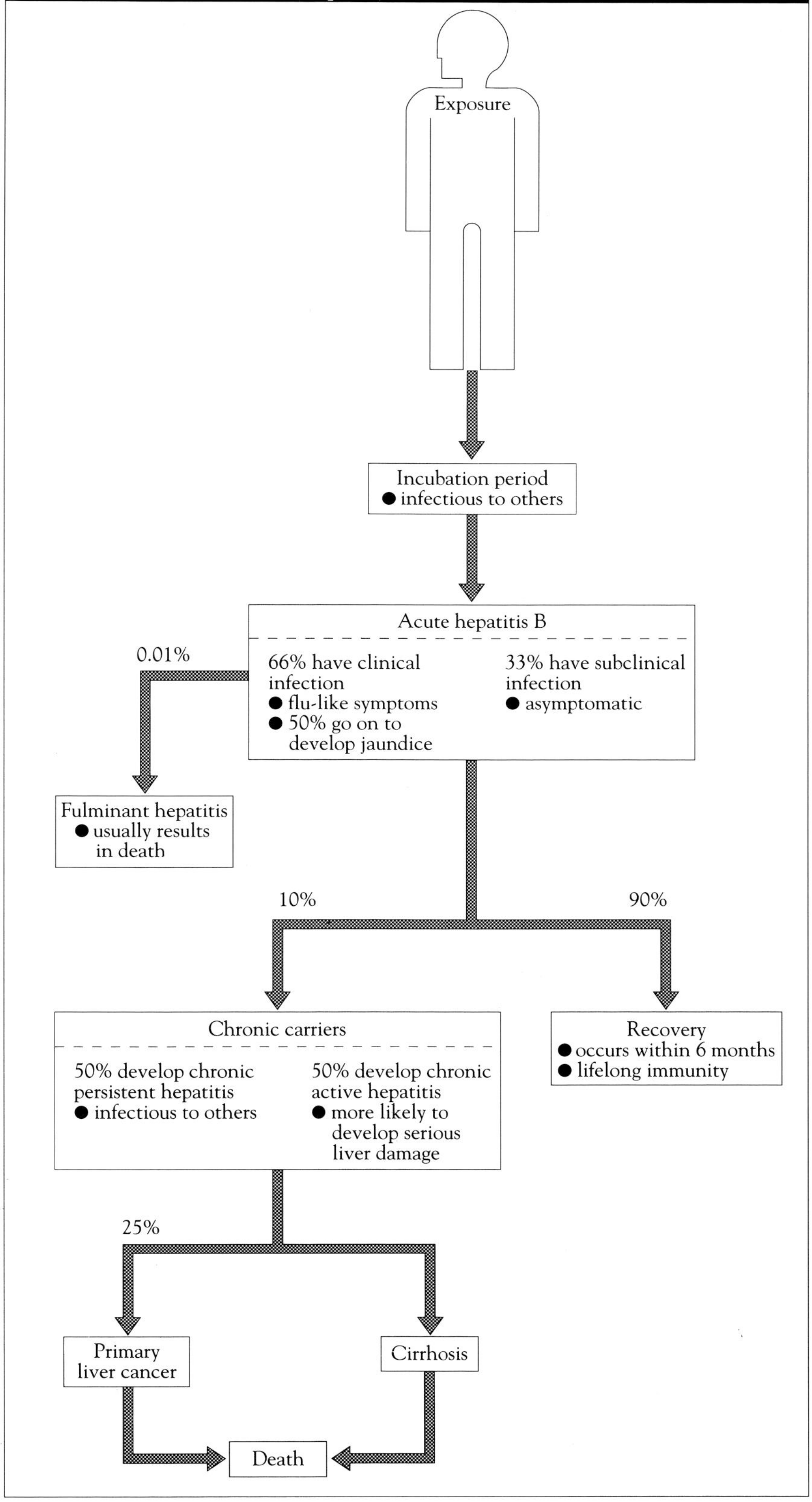

Figure 6.2: Clinical course of hepatitis B

the risks have been recognised, blood has been screened and staff have taken greater precautions. The introduction of effective hepatitis B vaccines means that the incidence of infection should now be virtually eliminated; staff at risk should be made aware of the risks and provided with the vaccine. New Department of Health guidelines stipulate that all health care workers undertaking exposure prone procedures, which could place patients at risk of infection by the hepatitis B virus (HBV), must show evidence of their immune status to hepatitis B. For most health care workers this will involve immunisation, with a satisfactory antibody response.[33]

In some people with infective hepatitis the disease is caused by other viruses such as the hepatitis C virus (HCV). Like hepatitis B, this virus is transmitted in blood, and anti-hepatitis C antibodies indicating previous infection, have been found in up to 5% of staff in renal dialysis units.[34,35] No vaccine is yet available for HCV (or HIV) and it is important that safe working practices are established, monitored and updated and that staff are fully trained in infection control practices. The small number of occupational exposures followed up so far suggest that the risk of infection may be about 3%.[36]

Human immunodeficiency virus (HIV)

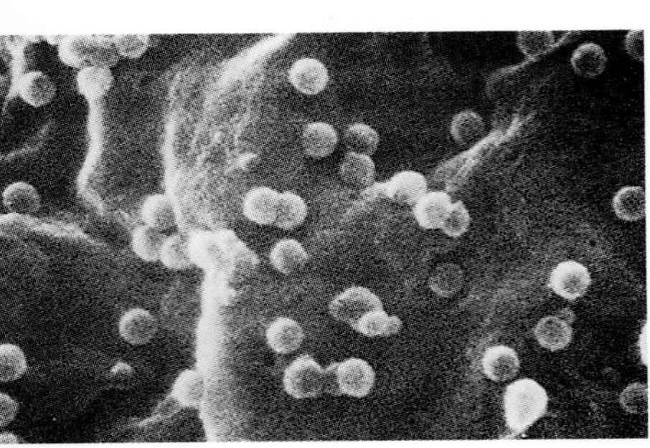

Human immunodeficiency virus (HIV) particles shown budding from cultured lymphocytes; (magnified approx. x 40,000)

Many of the measures, such as not resheathing needles and more effective instrument decontamination, which have helped reduce infection rates with hepatitis B, were introduced following concern over the transmission of HIV. Like hepatitis B, this virus is spread by blood-to-blood contact, although the risk of infection is much lower than with hepatitis B, ie. about 1 in 300 (0.3%). Fewer viral particles may be present than in the blood of HBV-infected patients, and it appears that a larger volume of blood is required to transmit HIV — such as from a deep penetrating injury with a hollow-bore needle, where patient blood is inoculated. If infection with HIV does occur it is much more likely to cause serious disease (acquired immune deficiency disease, (AIDS)) and mortality. Worldwide there are now 64 cases of documented occupationally acquired HIV infections in health care staff, with a further 118 cases presumed.[37]

The risk to patients of contracting HIV infection from health care workers or during medical procedures has proved to be of great concern to the general public. In five lookback exercises which have taken place in the UK, the total number of patients notified was 1801, of whom 689 are known to have been tested for HIV. All HIV tests were negative. All other retrospective studies worldwide of patients exposed to the potential risk of transmission of HIV during exposure prone procedures have failed to identify any who have become infected by this route. In the United States, the Centers for Disease Control and Prevention have found no evidence than any of the 19,036 persons tested following treatment by 57 HIV-infected health care workers were infected by this route.

In the light of current knowledge, the routine testing for HIV in health care workers performing exposure prone procedures as a measure to protect

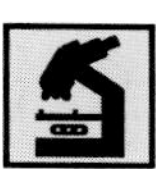

patients from infection is not justified. Any statutory policy, whether in the health care setting or not, which compels defined groups of individuals to be tested for HIV infection is discriminatory, interferes with an individuals rights and may deter those who are most in need of education and counselling from seeking advice. It is also not cost-effective.[38] Confidential, voluntary HIV testing should be available for health care workers, through a consultant led occupational health service and there should be clear careers guidance for health care workers infected with HBV or HIV.

Prions

The infectivity of prions ('slow viruses') has been highlighted recently by the epidemic of bovine spongiform encephalopathy (BSE) associated with cattle feeding on the remains of sheep infected with the scrapie virus.[39] Similar, transmissible, virus-like agents are responsible for Creutzfeldt-Jakob disease, a rare cause of dementia, in humans. These agents can contaminate neurosurgical and pathology equipment and are resistant to normal methods of disinfection and sterilisation. Creutzfeldt-Jakob disease has been known to be transmitted from patient-to-patient via contaminated brain electrodes, subcutaneous injections, and corneal implants.[40] Staff in neuropathology departments have occasionally developed the disease.[41] Although invasive neurosurgical procedures carry some risk of cross infection, the risk is thought to be very low.

Discussion

A variety of microbial hazards present risks to those in the health care environment at present, including infection from HIV and HBV and HCV. Vaccination is not available for HCV or HIV, so it is essential that staff are trained in infection control procedures. This training, along with the protection of staff and surveillance of procedures are the responsibility of

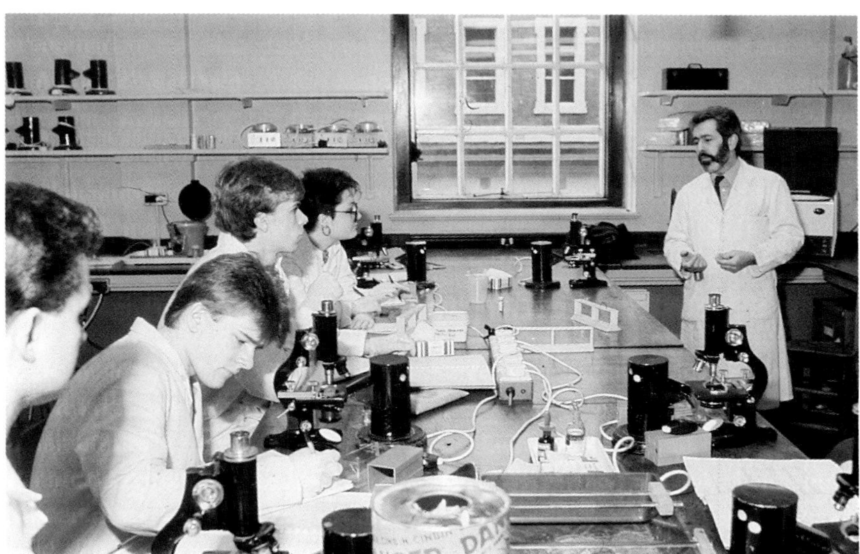

Health service employers should be required to provide immunisation for all staff and students who are in frequent contact with body fluids and sharps

hospital infection control committees. As vaccination is possible against HBV, health service employers should be *required* to provide immunisation for all staff and students who are in frequent contact with body fluids and sharps. Future developments in the field of genetic engineering may carry risks of microbial infection for scientific and hospital staff as discussed in Chapter 8, and new microbial hazards may arise in the future. With the development of effective infection control committees and occupational health services, infection control measures should enable future epidemics to be recognised early on, and dealt with effectively.

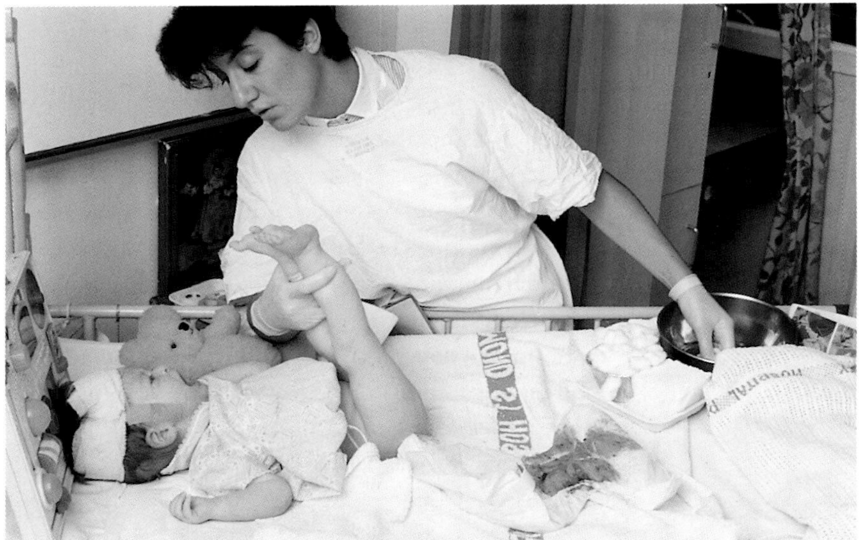

Prevention of virus transmission: it is essential that staff are trained in infection control procedures

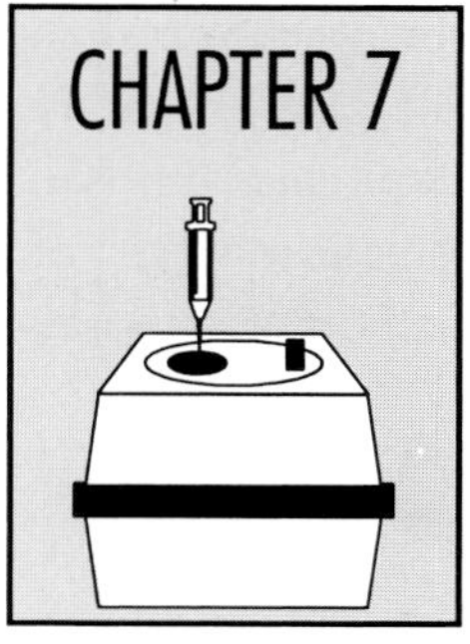

Clinical waste

In the majority of NHS hospitals, waste management, as a practice, does not exist; waste is treated simply as material that requires disposal. Until the early 1980s neither public nor politicians showed much interest in the potentially hazardous effects of waste materials produced by the health services or medical research establishments. Much of the material, now known as clinical waste, found its way onto municipal or commercial landfill sites or was burned in hospital incinerators. A series of widely publicised incidents, in which blood-stained dressings, used syringes and needles, tissues, and even cultures and pathological specimens discarded by laboratories, were found in public places and on leisure sites, brought the issue to the public's attention and caused revulsion and concern.[1]

The prominence of waste incinerators as landmarks, as well as the visual record of dark smoke, a sulphurous smell, or the appearance of charred pieces of paper in the air have no doubt contributed to the public's hostility to incineration. Understandably, it has been questioned whether these emissions might lead to the dispersion of heavy metals, grit, dust and other irritants and the production of toxic chemicals such as dioxins and furans.[2] For municipal incinerators used to destroy clinical waste, the use of internal conveyors and vibrating grates may lead to the incomplete destruction of micro-organisms. It is therefore possible that when an incinerator is overloaded, unburned or incompletely burned material carrying viable organisms could escape from the incinerator stack. It must be stressed, however, that there is no evidence of the health of operators or members of the public being affected by such emissions.

The present situation

Current practice in the majority of hospitals is to classify all waste from a 'clinical' area as 'clinical waste', irrespective of the hazard of that waste or

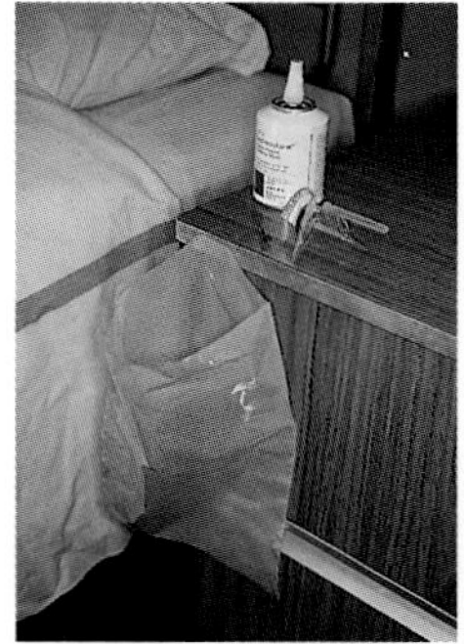
Only clinical waste should be disposed of in a yellow bag

the risks associated with it. The usual method of disposing of clinical waste is incineration, either on site in the hospital's own incinerator or at the incinerator belonging to another hospital nearby within the same district or region. At present, private waste disposal contractors are used occasionally when NHS plant fails or where there is a shortage of incineration capacity.

In general, there is no separation or segregation of waste in a clinical area; all waste is consigned to a yellow bag. In non-clinical areas, where non-clinical waste should be disposed of in black bags, the practice is such that most of this waste is still incinerated, either because black bags are transported to the waste disposal facility in the same vehicle as clinical waste, or because some administrative areas generate a small number of confidential documents and, for want of an alternative method of disposal, all of the waste produced is put into a yellow bag.

The present situation in context

In order to understand present waste management practices in the NHS, it is important to review the context in which they have developed. One of the most important factors in this respect was the possession of Crown immunity, whereby NHS incineration plants were exempt from prosecution under the statutory regulations governing municipal incinerators. Placing waste disposal facilities on hospital sites outside the law encouraged a culture in which investment into upgrading old plant or, indeed building new plant, was not an overriding priority. Years of under investment have lead to a situation where most of the plant existing in the NHS will not be able to comply with Environmental Protection Act (1990) standards by the deadline of 1995.

During a similar time-frame, there has been an increase in concern about certain viral infectious diseases such as HIV, and viral hepatitis. This epidemiological context has encouraged, and at times provided justification for, waste management practices and policies, that describe nothing more than incineration for the majority of waste produced on a hospital site. This practice is intimately related to the concurrent increase in the use of single-use disposable products. Again, the justification for their use has at times hinged on the spread of HIV and the risks of contracting hepatitis.

What is clinical waste?

At the time of the well publicised incidents of disposal by landfill of clinical waste authorities faced with demands for the resolution of this unsatisfactory state of affairs had problems in legally defining clinical waste. Although there were two published classifications of clinical waste,[3,4] no legal definition existed under The Control of Pollution Act (1974). The Government, in its response to the House of Commons Environment Committee Report on Toxic Waste confirmed the need for a 'consistent vocabulary' in the management of hazardous waste.[5] Eventually, clinical

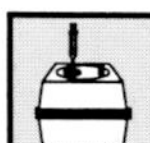

Legal definition of clinical waste

Any waste which consists wholly or partly of human or animal tissue, blood or any other body fluids, excretions, drugs or other pharmaceutical products, swabs or dressings, or syringes, needles or other sharp instruments, being waste, which unless rendered safe may prove hazardous to any person coming into contact with it; and any other waste arising from medical, nursing, dental, veterinary, pharmaceutical or similar practice, investigation, treatment, care, teaching or research, or the collection of blood for transfusion, being waste which may cause infection to any person coming into contact with it.

waste was defined legally under two Statutory Instruments.[6,7] The definition is given in the box on page 87.

Although these Regulations were issued under The Control of Pollution Act (1974) and The Environmental Protection Act (1990), the definitions relate to the effects on human health. The environment is also affected because any improper handling and disposal that affects health may also result in pollution. The term 'ecotoxic' has been coined for waste that is considered to pose a risk to the environment.

Regardless of the legal definitions of clinical waste, understanding at the workplace is vague. This is not surprising as what is disposed of as clinical waste may be at variance with the definition given in the Controlled Waste Regulations (1992) and waste staff may be asked to consign a wide range of waste products, unnecessarily, to clinical waste containers.

Classifications of clinical waste

A paper published by the Health and Safety Commission[8] and in general use in the UK classifies clinical waste in terms of the potential risks to health and safety (see box on page 88). These classifications (soon to be revised) list most, but not all, kinds of clinical waste.

Environmental pollution arises from the improper handling and disposal of clinical waste. In terms of environmental impact waste may be classified as:

(a) infectious;

(b) mechanically injurious;

(c) chemically toxic or noxious;

(d) aesthetically objectionable;

(e) any combinations of the above.

By assessing waste in terms of its environmental risks, safer and more efficient disposal systems can be designed.

Catgories of clinical waste (HSC 1993)

Group A
All human tissues, including blood (whether infected or not), animal carcasses and tissue from veterinary centres, hospitals or laboratories, and all related swabs and dressings. Waste materials where assessment indicates a risk to staff handling them, for example, from patients with infectious disease. Soiled surgical dressings, swabs and all other soiled waste from treatment areas.

Group B
Discarded syringes, needles, cartridges, broken glass and other sharp instruments.

Group C
Microbiological cultures and potentially infected waste from pathology departments (laboratory and postmortem rooms) and other clinical or research laboratories.

Group D
Certain pharmaceutical and chemical waste.

Group E
Items used to dispose of urine, faeces and other bodily secretions and excretions assessed as not falling within Group A. This includes used disposable bedpan liners, incontinence pads, stoma bags and urine containers.

Infectious waste

Infectious waste contains pathogenic micro-organisms (the term here includes viruses), any of which may be transmitted directly or indirectly to humans and animals. From wards and treatment centres it includes dressings, body fluids and excreta and the containers and disposable equipment used to collect them; hypodermic needles and syringes used to collect blood and fluids and administer medicaments; and disposable clothing and gloves. The most infectious kind of waste, which contains a wide variety and the largest number of pathogens, is generated by laboratories which concentrate the organisms by culture.

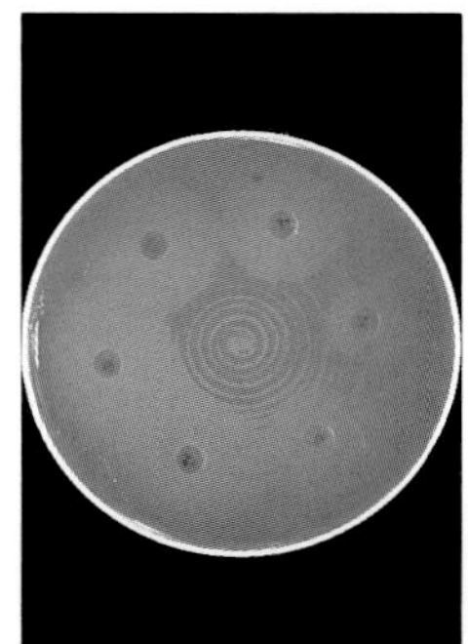

E. coli. *The most infectious kind of waste is generated by laboratories which concentrate organisms by culture*

'Sharps' and mechanically injurious waste

The most important components of this category of waste are 'sharps' and are defined as "...anything that can puncture the skin and may be contaminated with blood or other body fluid; this includes sharp bones as well as...hypodermic and suture needles and blades...".[9] Broken glass should be included within this category. Aerosol containers which may

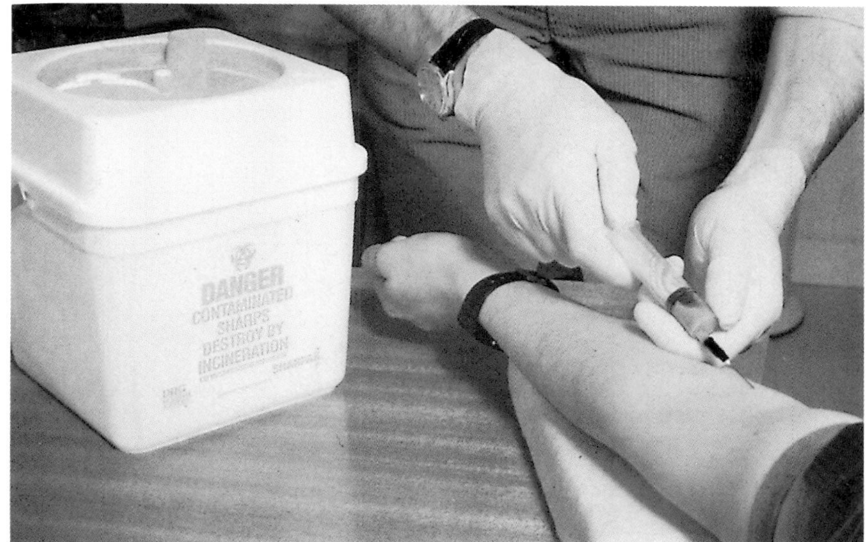

Immediately after use a needle should be dropped, while still attached to the syringe, into an impenetrable sharps disposal container

explode if handled roughly or exposed to heat are considered as mechanically injurious waste.

Sharps injury, especially from used needles, forms the most important route of infection for health care workers exposed to blood from hepatitis B positive patients. The epidemic of HIV has led to renewed concern among health care workers about the risks they face in hospital and clinical environments, HCV is likely to be readily transmitted in the same way.[10]

Most injuries are of two types; the first, many of which are preventable through the use of correct procedures and through training, occur during use of the syringe and needle and are typically self-inflicted wounds at the bedside or whilst preparing solutions for injection or during venepuncture. The second occur downstream away from the bedside and often involve another individual and an unidentifiable needle. These accidents may occur during clean-up after procedures, during needle disposal into overfilled containers or when staff encounter inappropriately discarded needles. In Central Sterile Supplies Departments (CSSDs) injuries may occur where staff sort dirty instruments by hand before cleaning. Treatment of used instruments by immersion in a detergent solution with ultrasound *before* sorting in CSSDs could reduce this risk. Other important sharps injuries may involve assistants helping at operations or during other clinical procedures when they are stuck with a needle or cut on the hand with a scalpel by a colleague. Even a single sharp (eg used needle) may present a risk, and particular attention should be paid to its safe disposal.

In 1983 the US Centres for Disease Control established guidelines for needle disposal,[11] which were adopted by the BMA in 1990. It was recommended that immediately after use, a needle should be dropped, whilst still attached to the syringe, into an impenetrable sharps disposal container at the bedside. Needles should not be recapped as up to 40% of all accidents involve resheathing or recapping the needle after use. The BMA issued detailed guidance on 'sharps' in 1990 in its *Code of Practice for the*

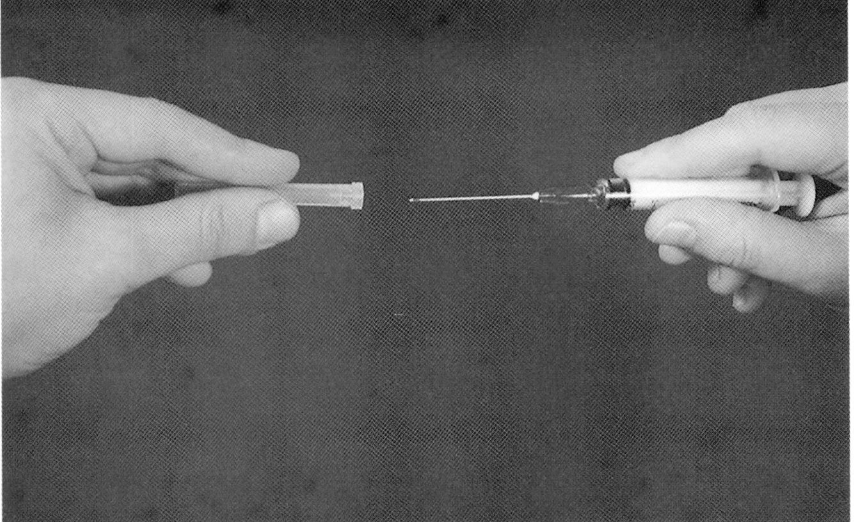

Up to 40% of all needlestick injuries involve resheathing or recapping the needle after use.

a) The health care worker aims the needle towards the resheathing cap and

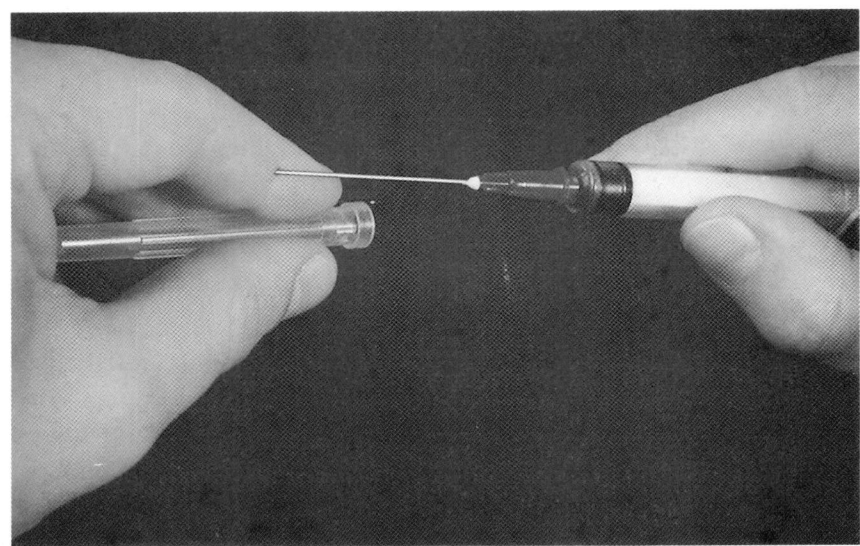

b) misses, jabbing the hand holding the cap

Safe Use and Disposal of Sharps.[12] However, guidance on not resheathing needles has been poorly followed in the intervening years.

Chemically toxic or noxious wastes and aesthetically objectional wastes

A distinction must be drawn for chemically toxic or noxious wastes between chemical substances that are used therapeutically or are administered for diagnostic purposes — namely pharmaceuticals and radionuclides — and those that are not so used, such as laboratory chemicals. The former are clinical waste, the latter are not and should be disposed of as hazardous or controlled wastes for which separate arrangements, under different regulations, are in force. Even among therapeutic and diagnostic substances a distinction should be made between the immediate residues of treatment or diagnosis and bulk pharmaceuticals that are out of date or no longer

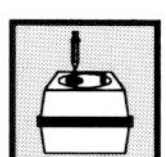

required. As with laboratory chemicals, these should not be included as clinical waste.

There are also wastes that while non-toxic before disposal may, become so during improper treatment. These are mainly plastics which, if not incinerated at appropriate temperatures, may produce pollutants and toxic substances such as dioxins.

In some of the unfortunate incidents reported, human tissues, including amputated tissue and placentas, were exposed on landfill sites. Aside from the potential hazards these might cause to people's health the public understandably condemned them as aesthetically objectionable. Clearly landfill is an unacceptable method of disposal for this category of clinical waste.

Collection and transport of clinical waste

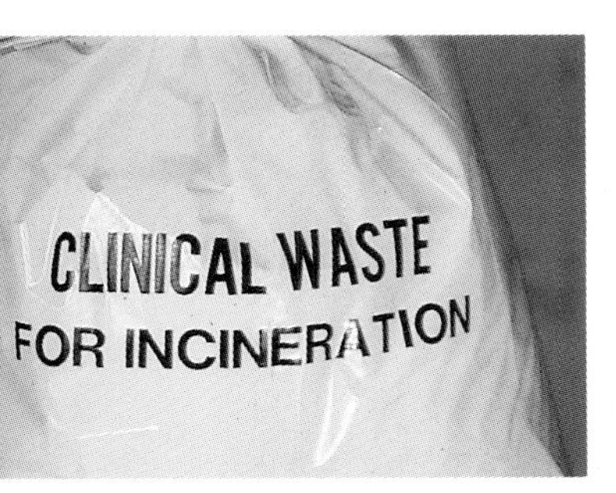

Plastic bags are unsuitable for amputations and other large items of surgical material

It is of considerable importance that the actual risks associated with the various components of the clinical waste stream generated in hospitals, at other health care sites, and in the community are assessed, to determine the waste management systems employed. Risk assessments can be used to inform any waste management policy and then guidance can be developed for the treatment and disposal of all wastes generated in the process of delivering health care.

Environmental contamination may occur between the generation of clinical waste and its ultimate disposal. In the UK clinical waste is usually placed in yellow plastic bags,[13] or in the case of sharps, in specially constructed plastic containers, also coloured yellow, and of a specified nature.[14] Unless handled with care, however, plastic bags may burst and scatter their contents at any time during their transportation which include: generation point to hospital collection site; hospital collection site to local authority or commercial transfer station, and transfer station to incinerator or landfill site. Where clinical waste is collected and processed by specialist commercial organisations, the practice is to place batches of plastic bags in more robust containers; these may be either 'one-trip' heavy duty card containers or rigid plastic ones that can be disinfected and cleaned before reuse. Plastic bags are unsuitable for amputations and other large items of surgical material; some hospitals are now using more rigid containers. On mainland Europe more substantial primary containers are often used instead of plastic bags, and some European authorities believe that these should replace the plastic bags now used in the UK.

Municipal solid waste from domestic or commercial premises is often mechanically compressed (compacted) in the collection vehicles. This process ruptures plastic bags, leads to leakage of fluid contents and dispersal of air-borne micro-organisms. This process can be hazardous if applied to clinical waste. Several official bodies as well as the Health and Safety Commission[15] issue advice on the safe handling of clinical waste. These include the Department of the Environment,[16] the London Waste Regulation Authority[17,18] and the National Association of Waste Disposal Contractors.[19]

This advice covers the types of bulk containers and methods for moving and storing them. This legislation comprises The Control of Pollution Act (1974) and The Environmental Protection Act (1990).

Options for disposal

At present, most clinical waste is either incinerated or disposed of in landfill sites, although some is autoclaved first. Different treatment technologies are being developed which may change the future of decontamination and disposal. It is rare, however, that any method proves entirely problem free, and current experiments in Europe should be monitored.

Incineration

Objections to incineration are largely based on the poor performance and objectionable emissions of many hospital incinerators, a situation publicised by the National Clean Air Association.[20] There is also a fear that dioxins and other toxic substances may be released when certain plastics and other substances are incinerated. Ash residues have also been suspected of causing problems, sometimes with good reason.[21] The new generation of efficient incinerators with their continuous automatic monitoring should eliminate such risks on scientific and technical grounds. The high temperatures, adequate mixing and retention times achieved, and the filtration and scrubbing of the effluent, prevent the emission of toxic substances or micro-organisms. Emissions from these incinerators must comply with standard codes of practice, guidelines and regulations[22] and various Guidance Notes and EC Directives.[23-26] Furthermore, the ash residues are treated as controlled waste and disposed of accordingly.

The National Health and Community Care Act (1990) lifted Crown immunity from hospital premises. This Act and other impending legislation led to health authorities decommissioning many unsatisfactory incinerators that could not be upgraded to meet national standards.[27-31]

Unfortunately, the result was that neither hospitals nor the commercial sector had sufficient incinerators and those in operation were unevenly distributed throughout the UK in relation to the sources of clinical waste.[32,33] Refurbishing incinerators is expensive and the installation of new plant even more costly. Moreover, waste disposal costs are set to increase for the foreseeable future as environmental legislation, particularly that governing waste disposal, becomes more stringent. With the loss of Crown immunity occurring conjointly with the advent of the Environmental Protection Act (1990), all incinerator plants in the NHS will need to comply with Environmental Protection Act (1990) standards by the deadline of 1995. However, in 1995 more stringent emission standards will come into operation resulting in a further number of hospital incinerators having to close. A national survey of clinical waste carried out by the Institution of Environmental Health Officers in 1992 confirmed that many hospitals will fail to meet these standards and an anticipated shortfall in incineration

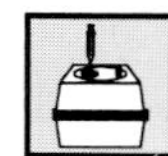

capacity can be expected.[34] The net result will be that clinical waste from NHS hospitals will have to be sent to either private waste disposal contractors or municipal incinerators, to be disposed of at market prices. This could be a costly requirement if the present waste management practices and policies are retained.

A draft EC Directive states that clinical waste should not be disposed of in landfill sites, and the UK Government and the European Community are committed to incinerating all clinical waste by 1995.[35] Apart from the cost and technical problems, however, there remains the problem of convincing the public that incinerators, however sophisticated, are safe. The restrictions on access to information in the public domain in the UK in comparison with other European and US authorities does little to allay the publics concerns.

Landfill disposal

Most UK authorities now oppose the disposal of clinical waste on landfill sites[36,37] and as highlighted earlier the UK Government and European Community are committed to incinerating all clinical waste by 1995.[38] However, until sufficient incineration facilities are available, some landfill disposal of clinical waste will continue. Objections to the landfill disposal of clinical waste are based on the risk of transmission to individuals of pathogenic micro-organisms, either directly by contact, or indirectly by insect and animal vectors and the pollution of water supplies. A BMA report on hazardous waste and human health[39] concluded that there was a lack of up-to-date research into landfill and that there was inadequate environmental monitoring of sites and standards of quality control.

Autoclaving (steam sterilisation)

Some clinical waste from hospital wards and departments may be autoclaved, usually at 121°C for 30 minutes. If properly controlled, this method results in 'safe', namely non-infectious, waste but it does not reduce the bulk. Some of the material is still recognisable as clinical waste and aesthetically unacceptable to the public.

Infectious waste from microbiological and biomedical laboratories, consisting of pathological specimens and cultures should be autoclaved before it leaves the laboratory premises. This is standard, good microbiological practice.[40,41] It is also implied in a report from the Advisory Committee on Dangerous Pathogens[42] which states, "all waste materials must be safe before disposal or removal to the incinerator." Unfortunately, recent official advice in the Health Services Advisory Committee document, *Safe Working and the Prevention of Infection in Clinical Laboratories,*[43] still permits such highly infectious waste to leave laboratories untreated en route to incinerators which may be some distance away "if it is not reasonably practicable to autoclave waste...". Despite the caveats and existing regulations this means that there is a considerable risk of accidental dispersion leading to pollution and the spread of infection. As autoclaves are essential equipment in all reputable microbiological laboratories this waste could be made safe by autoclaving before it is removed for final disposal, preferably by incineration.

Novel methods of disposal

These include maceration, with or without chemical disinfection, and then disposal via the public sewer; exposure to ionising radiation; or treatment with microwaves. Maceration may generate aerosols, exposing operators to infection or the inhalation of toxic substances, including any disinfectant used, and may affect sewage disposal. This method may be used for small volumes of clinical waste such as tissues, but only after consultation with the water companies. Microwave treatment techniques have been licensed for use in Pembrokeshire NHS Trust, although ionising radiation technology is still at a developmental stage. Even if this method is successful, although the waste may be made 'safe' there will still be the problem of final disposal. Like the autoclaving of infectious laboratory waste, microwave treatment may prove a useful interim measure if the final disposal site is a long way from where the waste originates.

Domestic or clinical waste

Modern 'hygiene' technology, together with public awareness of environmental pollution and other health hazards, especially about HIV, hepatitis B and diarrhoeal diseases, have prompted concerns about the disposal of used sanitary towels, tampons and disposable nappies. Questions centre on the infectious hazards posed by these articles and whether they qualify as clinical waste or as domestic (municipal solid) waste.

The situation in the home differs from that in hospitals and other health care environments since the quantity of waste involved is usually very small. Much of this will be produced and handled only by the patient or the family, in circumstances outside the scope of the Health and Safety at Work etc Act (1974). However, at times health care professionals, such as community nurses, will be treating the patient in the home and will have to deal with clinical waste. Current guidance from the HSC states that it is the duty of the health care worker's employer to ensure that clinical waste generated as a result of such home treatment is disposed of safely. Health care workers themselves also have duties under the Health and Safety at Work etc Act (1974) and the Environmental Protection Act (1990) to ensure safe and proper disposal. Disposal should be via employers' own systems, or by special arrangement with the local authority. Clinical waste collected in this way should not enter the domestic waste system.[44] However, further guidance is anticipated from the Department of the Environment. This may give the health care worker the responsibility to decide whether the waste generated from formal health care in the home poses sufficient risk to require disposal as clinical waste.

Where this waste originates in public conveniences or at premises where they are collected by the local authority then that authority has a choice:

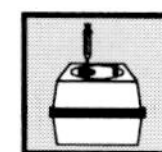

incineration or landfill. Since the bins in public lavatories and business premises for immediate disposal of hygiene products contain disinfectant the waste might reasonably be described as safe. Unfortunately, this is illusory because the disinfectant, even if effective and in the correct concentration, may never come into contact with the waste. The sight of blood may upset some people, who equate its presence with infection, and, indeed, menstrual blood may contain the HIV and hepatitis viruses. As for nappies, more diarrhoeal diseases occur in the home than in hospitals.

At present, there is a strategic shift towards providing care for patients in the community. Hospital-at-home schemes are being developed particularly for certain groups of patients such as children and the elderly. Indeed, in the Strategic Plan for the Oxford Regional Health Authority, a target has been set for 16,000 more domiciliary visits a year for each of the five years of the plan. In meeting these targets the problem of the generation, collection, transportation, treatment and final disposal of clinical waste in the community needs to be solved, and this will have cost implications. However, studies are being planned that will evaluate the problems of generating clinical waste in the community, and try to identify appropriate ways of solving them.

Economic issues

By failing to differentiate between different kinds of waste, the NHS spends unnecessary resources on inappropriately incinerating domestic waste under the guise of clinical waste. It is difficult to quantify the costs involved as there are no hard data on which to base the calculations, only best estimates. If the tonnage for the amount of clinical waste produced by the NHS in 1992 as reported by the National Society for the Protection of Clean Air (1992) is taken and then halved, (the current and generally accepted estimate is that 50% of the clinical waste sent for incineration is actually domestic waste) and then multiplied by £200, (the 1993 average unit cost of incinerating a tonne of clinical waste), the NHS could be spending from £56-£70 million a year on inappropriate incineration as the result of practices and policies that are in urgent need of reappraisal.

Waste minimisation

Since there is widespread anxiety about the volume of clinical waste and its impact on the environment, waste minimisation strategies should be considered.[45,46] In Germany 10 times less clinical waste per capita is generated than in the United Kingdom due to differences in clinical practice and waste categorisation.[47] In Germany the infectious status of any patient entering a hospital site is ascertained, and it is only if a patient is carrying an infection that the waste is designated and treated as clinical. Furthermore, waste is segregated according to the risk it presents. Only those wastes assessed to be of risk are incinerated as clinical waste. Both in the UK and the USA infection control is more stringent. Although medical practice is based on good history-taking and the examination of symptoms and signs for diagnosis it is not necessarily known whether a patient is infectious. To minimise the risk of cross infection, 'universal precautions' are increasingly applied, treating all patients as if they were infectious; hence, the much greater volume of clinical waste.

The use of disposable items also leads to increased levels of waste and it should be considered whether disposable items could safely be replaced with reusable ones. Arguments against reusable items include the risk that they may not be properly sterilised and so put patients at risk. The advent of AIDS and the risks of hepatitis infection have increased such fears.

Barriers to change

It is clear that the present waste disposal practices within the NHS are unsustainable, not just in environmental terms but also in terms of the potential drain on resources. Unfortunately, there are several significant barriers to change:

- **Little central impetus or guidance**
  Apart from an internal document produced for the Department of Health in the latter half of 1990 (to coincide with the impending loss of Crown immunity), there has been little co-ordinated central guidance on the issue of waste management in the NHS. The Estates Directorate of the Department of Health, which usually gave advice on this and related issues, now receives no direct government funding and undertakes work on a consultancy basis.

  Other bodies or government departments which work in the area of clinical waste are the Department of the Environment, which at the time of writing is conducting a revision of Waste Management Paper No. 25 on Clinical Waste, and the Health Service Advisory Group of the Health and Safety Executive, which issued new guidelines for the safe disposal of clinical waste in 1992.

- **NHS reforms**
  The conversion of directly managed units into NHS trusts which are responsible for their own budgets and compete for business has divided the NHS. The application of market forces in a drive to improve the quality and value for money of health care has had other effects. There is a tendency to a more isolationist approach, such that if one trust were to identify significant cost savings it may not share that information with other trusts competing to provide clinical services. The result is a reduction in the degree of liaison, networking and information-sharing that takes place in the NHS.

- **Environmental management systems are not regarded as a core priority in the NHS**
  Environmental management systems, particularly those relating to waste management, are not regarded as a core priority, ie not directly

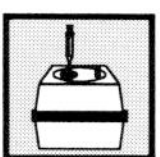

related to patient care. As such, the degree of support senior managers might give to the development of such systems is negligible.

- **The low and declining level of expertise**
  Waste disposal is normally the province of the Estates Department. However, the estates function is increasingly being seen as a non-core service within health care, with consequent redundancies in this area of work. The prevailing management style is to have 'informed client' status, which means that the client, in this case the NHS, is informed enough to buy the non-core services from external contractors as appropriate. Unfortunately, there are some areas of work for which services have to be bought-in, that require considerable knowledge and a sophisticated level of understanding. This applies to waste management and the appropriate handling and disposal of clinical and toxic wastes. The low and declining level of expertise within the estates function is, therefore, of concern.

- **Cost of investment**
  When the NHS lost Crown immunity in 1991 and became subject to the law, no ring-fenced monies were made available for either upgrading existing or building new incinerator plant to comply with the standards required by the Environmental Protection Act (1990). Without ring-fenced money the scale of investment required was too great for most sites operating an incinerator to undertake given their history of under investment during the possession of Crown immunity and the necessity for spending resources on patient care.

- **Lack of baseline data**
  It is difficult to implement and evaluate different waste management systems when the data available to work from are scarce and sometimes of poor quality. It is not known exactly how much waste the NHS generates, whether at health care sites or in the community, or indeed the proportion of the various components within the waste stream and from which specialties these wastes are generated. Of course, there are many estimates but unfortunately no firm basis for most of them. This lack of data is also a hindrance when arguing for change as any statements are open to challenge.

Discussion

Fortunately, during the past decade legislation has been directed at what microbiologists call 'containment'; the encapsulation of hazardous material so that it does not 'escape' between where it originates and its site of destruction. Incineration in modern plant that uses state-of-the-art technology is the preferred method of preventing environmental pollution from the rising volume of clinical waste. Resources should therefore be earmarked to ensure a national network of modern incinerators accessible by all health care units producing clinical waste. This should be backed by appropriate national regulations that include regular monitoring.

The NHS should aim to develop appropriate waste management systems for all the waste arising from health care in whatever setting, based on risk assessments of the relevant components of the various waste streams. 'Appropriate' is a key word, because at present the NHS may be spending money inappropriately on a form of waste disposal for certain wastes that do not need to be treated in a particular way; conversely, the NHS may not be spending enough money on the appropriate disposal of some of the more toxic wastes it generates. Waste management systems may need to be co-ordinated at a regional or national strategic level. At present, work is being undertaken within Oxford Regional Health Authority that could provide the baseline data from which many of the questions posed here could be answered. This work has also stimulated an opening of the debate about the true risks of clinical waste, not only to staff and patients, but also to the general public and the environment.

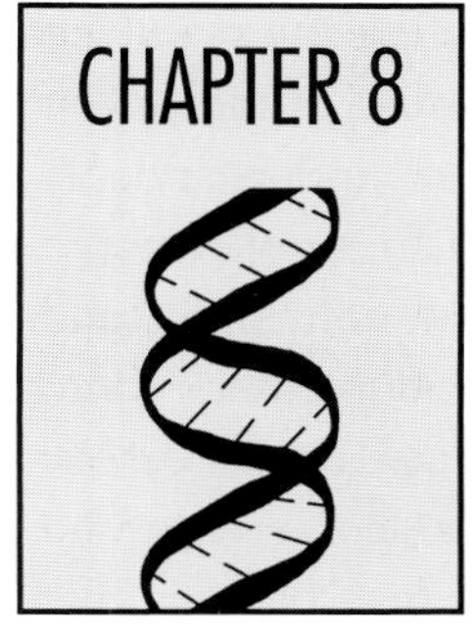

CHAPTER 8

Genetic modification

From Darwin's initial attempts to explain evolution in terms of natural selection and Mendel's discovery of the rudiments of how inheritance works through individual genes, we have progressed to a detailed knowledge of the make-up and functioning of a large proportion of the genetic material in man and other organisms. As the basic structure of genetic material is common to all known life, and genes are responsible for determining most of the characteristics which make us as we are, they are central to life itself. Genes are responsible for determining characteristics such as body shape, hair and eye colour, and they may help to determine much of our peculiarly human behaviour. Differences in the information carried in genes determine differences between biological species, so that, for example, animals develop differently from each other and from much simpler forms of life such as bacteria and plants.

Genetic modification is the artificial modification of the structure or expression of genes. Control of genetic material, the code that dictates the nature of life of plants and animals, could provide us with a potentially very powerful tool, giving some control over life and death. Our control of this code could enable the production of plants and animals with particular characteristics, including resistance to a disease. In short, the characteristics important in life could be dictated to nature. The benefits of this are easily imagined, and some have already been realised, but there are hazards too.

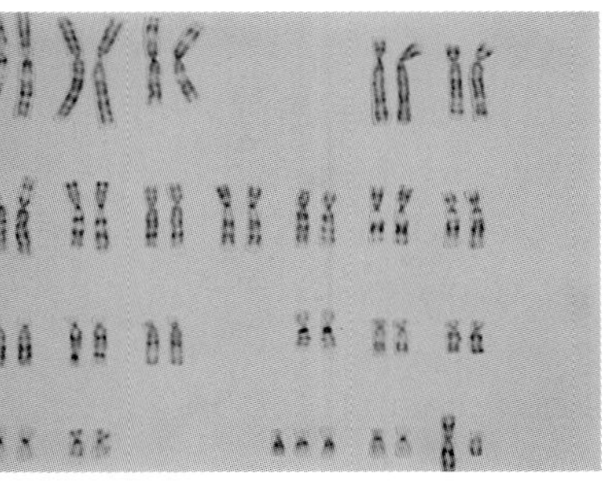

This chorionic villus sample has revealed that the foetus has Down's syndrome. The normal human complement of chromosomes is 23 pairs, but those with Down's syndrome have an extra chromosome (see bottom row seventh chromosome from right)

Genetic engineering has been used for centuries, firstly as selection by breeders and latterly as deliberately induced mutations of yeasts, flowers, antibiotic producing organisms etc. Recent advances in genetic modification techniques have increased the potency and selectivity of our ability to produce genetic changes. Today, genetic modification is applied in agriculture, in the pharmaceutical industry and is now being applied in medicine, where the possibilities of genetic modification are being explored. Already several drugs and vaccines have been produced using genetically modified micro-organisms. A potential objective is the correction of inherited genetic diseases and it may prove possible to produce human proteins and even complete 'human' organs within other animals. Genetically modified animals could also provide models for investigating human disease.

Inevitably there will be a demand for genetic modification and the technique will become widespread. One consequence will be that some of the manufactured genes will enter the environment, where they will no longer be easily monitored and controlled. Perhaps because of the power that genetic modification has to change life, people are understandably worried about any loss of control over novel genes, which, once released into the environment, may spread between organisms with unintended and unforeseen consequences. A gene to produce a useful product inserted into a bacteria could produce a new type of disease if the gene (or the genetic rearrangement) were pathogenic, and the bacteria were able to escape and then either infect humans or transfer the relevant gene to a bacteria that does infect humans. In nature, the transfer of genetic material between bacteria is relatively commonplace. Certain genes used constructively to promote growth in one organism may cause unrestrained growth in another, with harmful consequences.

Clearly, this powerful tool needs careful control to obtain optimum benefits. The potential for benefit in medicine and in other areas is enormous, but so is the potential for harm. In this section we discuss some of the present and possible future applications of genetic modification in medicine, and we try to estimate the potential for environmental harm that could be a consequence of these techniques. This chapter briefly reviews existing controls on genetic modification in the UK; the science and ethics of genetic technology have been covered extensively in a prior BMA publication *Our Genetic Future.*[1]

Applications involving modification of micro-organisms

Micro-organisms, usually bacteria, have been used widely in genetic modification studies. They are readily available, easily grown, and reproduce rapidly so allowing evolutionary changes to be detected quickly, and exist in very many species and strains. A vast library of pre-existing genes is available to be exploited. Micro-organisms have genes which are relatively easily modified, and nature has several established methods for removing or inserting genetic material which can usefully be harnessed by scientists. As such, they are ideal for genetic modification and also provide a convenient and productive method for expressing useful genes commercially because of their rapid reproduction. In the process these organisms produce great quantities of a gene product. They have thus been widely used for investigating the principles of genetics, and have quickly been adopted for some of the first commercial medical applications of genetic modification.

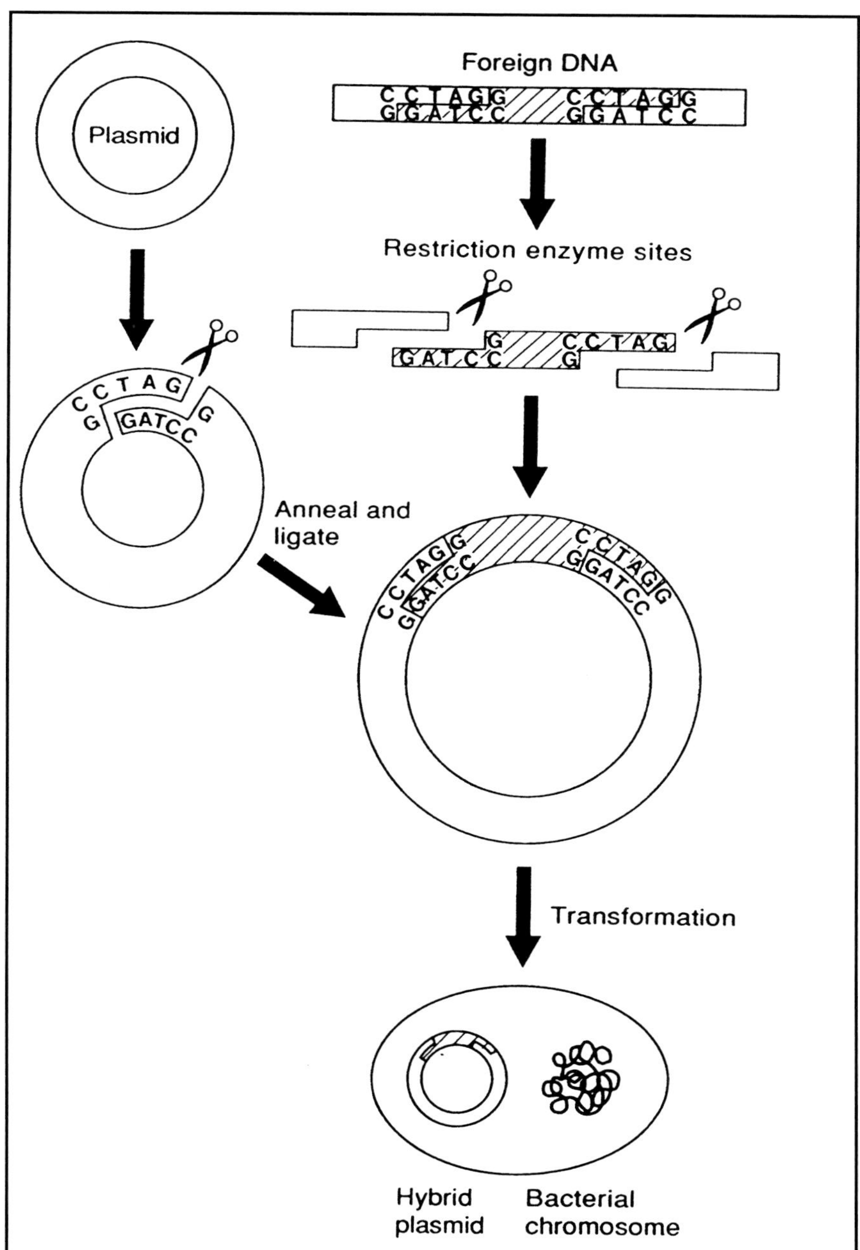

Figure 8.1: Foreign DNA is inserted into a vector - here a plasmid, which is then incorporated into the bacterial nucleus. Once inside the vector, the foreign DNA replicates every time the cell divides. Using this principle bacteria can be used to produce a range of human hormones and antibiotics

Pharmaceuticals

Extraction of the antibiotic penicillin from the fungus *Penicillium notatum* was an early application of micro-organisms in medicine. Initially discovered by Alexander Fleming occurring naturally in bacterial cultures, thanks to the alertness of other investigators, the fungus was soon being cultured on a commercial scale when its value in treating infections was confirmed. Researchers soon realised that by modifying culture conditions, and by selecting the 'best' strains, production of the required product could be optimised. They soon learnt, too, that by irradiating micro-organisms the incidence of genetic mutations could be increased, thus increasing the

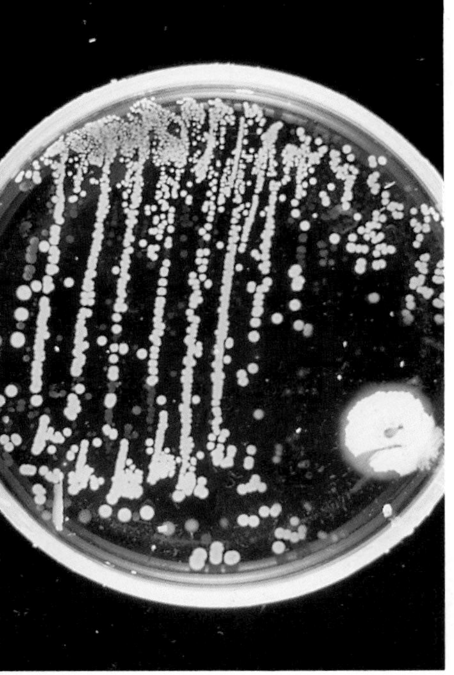

A reconstruction of Fleming's Penicillium notatum *culture: the large white spot on the right is the* penicillium *which has killed surrounding bacteria*

chances of producing a new and beneficial characteristic — an early if unsophisticated form of genetic modification. The gene for the production of penicillin already existed in *P. notatum* at the time of the fungus's discovery. But once the techniques for refining drugs produced from culture of micro-organisms had been perfected the potential for future use was soon obvious, provided that the micro-organisms could be made to produce the appropriate products. Modern techniques of genetic modification should, of course, allow the programming of micro-organisms to produce the required products using similar techniques of culture and purification.

For many years insulin used in treating diabetes was extracted from the pancreatic tissue of slaughtered cattle and pigs. The pancreas of the dead animals had to be collected and processed quickly to ensure the best yield of insulin, but the insulin produced differed from human insulin in some of its constituent amino acids and this could cause problems in treatment. By inserting the gene for human insulin into microbes in an appropriate way, and culturing them in large amounts, large quantities of insulin identical in its amino acid make-up to human insulin can now be produced much more cheaply and conveniently than previously. Although some patients experience problems of hypoglycaemia during the switch over from non-human to human insulin, this method of producing insulin is very successful and has now almost replaced the use of insulin extracted from cattle and pigs.

Several other products are produced in this way, so avoiding the need for laborious extraction and purification from dead tissue. Human growth hormone, and some other hormones were previously prepared by extraction from cadaveric human pituitary glands. Not only was this time consuming and unpleasant work, but it involved a risk of transmitting infection from donor to recipient. Several people given cadaveric human growth hormone subsequently died from Creutzfeldt Jakob disease, a prion disease of the human brain, almost certainly transmitted to the victim with the hormone.[2] Concern has arisen over a similar risk arising from past use of cadaveric human pituitary hormones in the treatment of infertility.[3] Human growth hormone is now produced using genetically modified bacteria, so avoiding

Some genetically produced substances used in the treatment of diseases[4]

- Interferon for the treatment of viral hepatitis
- Erythropoietin for the treatment of anaemia
- Human luteinising hormone for the treatment of infertility
- Tissue plasminogen activator for the treatment of heart disease and for thrombus dissolution in peripheral vascular disease
- Alpha-1-antitrypsin for the treatment of emphysema
- Human growth hormone for the treatment of retarded growth

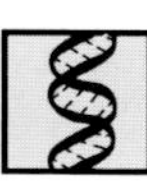

the risk of transmission of this disease. Some of the diverse range of products produced in this way and the diseases for which they are used are given in the box on page 102.

The bacterium most commonly used in genetically engineered therapeutic products is *Escherichia coli*, a commensal organism which normally colonises sections of the human gut, and is usually — though not always — harmless in that environment. Since the bacteria has to be confined in a culture vessel, the culture medium is usually sterilised before disposal. Furthermore, as the bacterium used is a 'normal compañion' of man, the risks of human contamination by a genetically engineered variant are thought to be low. However, we cannot afford to be complacent, since the risks of inadvertent release of these altered micro-organisms will still be present (and will increase as this production technique is more frequently used). Despite their commensal nature *E coli*, and probably any other micro-organisms used in the same way, can cause disease in humans — usually those whose body defences have been weakened — with *E coli*, a common cause of urinary tract infections. So the pathogenicity of a bacterium could be inadvertently enhanced in some unexpected way by the genetic modification which makes it useful.[5]

Vaccines

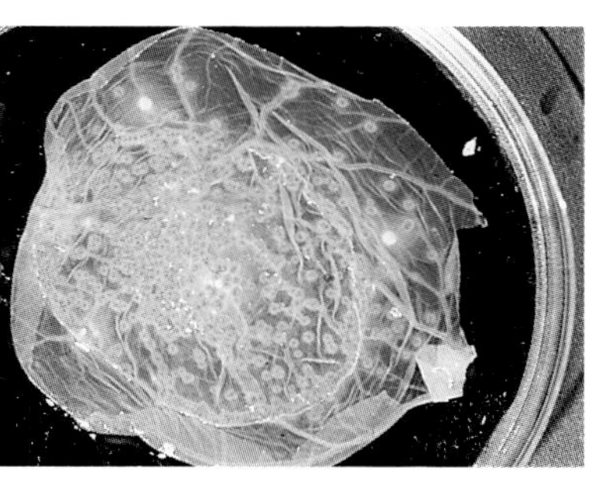

Egg culture of cowpox: Edward Jenner produced the first vaccine by inoculating volunteers with cowpox which successfully protected them against smallpox,

Two hundred years ago Jenner produced the first vaccine by inoculating volunteers with cowpox exudate through their skin and this protected them against smallpox. The natural existence of a safe immunising agent such as cowpox is exceptional, and it was Pasteur who subsequently developed a technique for reducing the pathogenicity of micro-organisms so that they could then be used for inoculation in the same way. Killed vaccines are also used, and several now consist only of the relevant fragments of a micro-organism. These are sufficient to allow it to be recognised as a foreign agent (antigen) and consequently confer some immunity against the natural disease. Most people in the UK have been immunised against the common childhood diseases and realise the benefits of this method of preventing certain infectious diseases.

Vaccination induces an immune response to the fragment or whole micro-organism which stimulates the production of defensive antibodies in the individual. Thereafter, if rechallenged with the same antigen, the body can respond quickly by producing antibodies, thus preventing the micro-organism establishing itself within the host and causing disease. Vaccines offer two ways of using genetic modification. Firstly, several vaccines can be produced in a similar way to the production of pharmaceutical products discussed above. The relevant gene for production of the antigen required to confer immunity in the host is inserted into an appropriate micro-organism. These are then cultured to produce the antigen, which is purified to produce a vaccine. Vaccines for hepatitis B, tetanus and diphtheria are already produced in this way.[6] Secondly, there are instances where the use of a live vaccine is more effective than a dead one. The Sabin polio vaccine used in the UK is an attenuated live vaccine, consisting of polio virus which has been altered so that it cannot cause disease. The advantage of using a live virus lies in the fact that it closely simulates the normal virus in its effect on the body, inducing a longer lasting and hence more protective immunity than the dead vaccine. Furthermore, it spreads to some extent from immunised individuals into the community thus increasing the level of immunity among that community and replacing in part the virulent 'wild' virus.

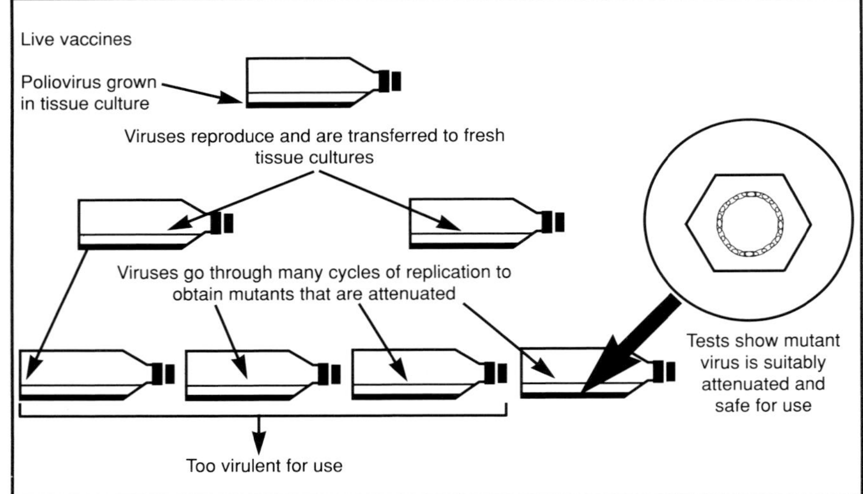

Figure 8.2: The Sabin polio vaccine used in the UK is an attenuated live vaccine, consisting of polio virus which has been altered so that it induces immunity without causing disease

Genetic modification is a precise tool for modifying live vaccines. Either the pathogenic micro-organism can be modified by removing the genes responsible for its virulence, or genes producing antigens from the micro-organism can be inserted into a harmless vector organism which can then be used to deliver the vaccine in an appropriate way. Taking this principle a stage further, one carrier could be made to produce the antigens which allow the body to develop immunity to a whole range of pathogenic micro-organisms. *Salmonella typhimurium*, a bacterium which causes food poisoning has been disabled in this way, the genes coding for certain enzymes being removed so that it dies within a few days of release, but not before it has provoked immunity without, causing disease. The vaccinia or cowpox virus has also been used as a carrier for some antigens. Genes from the viruses causing hepatitis B, rabies, and several other diseases have been inserted into the vaccinia virus.

This use of genetically modified micro-organisms means that they will pass into the environment. Although we are primarily concerned here with humans, the same techniques are also likely to be used for various animal and plant diseases, resulting in other genetically manipulated micro-organisms being released into the environment. Mostly, their escape will be inconsequential as they do not cause disease, nor are they likely to persist in competition with wild varieties of the same micro-organism. Circumstances may occur, however, when these altered micro-organisms could cause harm.

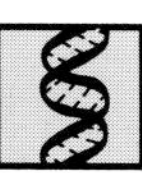

Release of genetically modified micro-organisms into the environment

The use of genetically modified micro-organisms has such potential advantages in medicine and a host of other fields that they will almost certainly be widely employed. Non-pathogenic bacteria will generally be used, and with proper controls are unlikely to be a threat to man or his environment. Commonly, culture medium is sterilised before disposal, and so in routine use the micro-organisms should have little environmental effect, although the disposal of large quantities of nutrient rich culture media may have unexpected effects in local rivers, etc. Accidental release of micro-organisms can occur, and the consequences would depend on several factors, including the type of organism, the site, route of release and proximity to centres of population, etc.

Large numbers of micro-organisms have for many years been released into the environment from activities such as sewage disposal and brewing. However, great care will be necessary when genetically modified micro-organisms are deliberately released into the environment as live vaccines or as carriers of foreign antigens. Precautions will be essential to minimise the risks inherent in this, including the use of disabled or normally non-pathogenic micro-organisms. Even so, several normally harmless micro-organisms can cause disease in certain circumstances. One example already noted is *E coli*, which can infect the urinary tract. The vaccinia virus, too, is potentially pathogenic, particularly for those individuals whose immune systems have been suppressed, for example, patients who have had an organ transplant and are on immunosuppressant drugs to prevent rejection, patients taking steroids for a variety of disorders, and people suffering from leukaemia or AIDS.

We can take further precautions to increase the margin of safety. Micro-organisms with a particular nutritional requirement can be used so that prolonged survival in the environment is impossible. Alternatively, small scale, controlled releases can be carried out initially so that the effect of the micro-organism can be studied, and appropriate corrective action taken if there are adverse consequences. Even with all these precautions we have

Uncertainty about consequences of genetic modification of micro-organisms

Bacteria and other micro-organisms can exchange genetic material among themselves with unrivalled promiscuity, sometimes in unforeseen ways and with unpredictable consequences. The speed of reproduction and the pace of evolution in their world can be rapid, so that any new gene that confers benefits to host organism could quickly become widespread. We must understand that the release of genetically modified micro-organisms will always entail uncertainty about the consequences.

to accept that releasing these micro-organisms into the environment means that we lose control over them. (see box on page 105)

Genetic modification in animals

The genetic modification of animals has been practised for many years and offers great potential benefits, medicine is one beneficiary. Animals may be bred in certain ways to produce valuable characteristics, for example, sheep with a particular type of fleece or cattle with a high milk yield. The new technology for directly manipulating genetic material will allow this selection process to be more precisely targeted, but otherwise the principle is little different in effect to established breeding techniques. Taken with the parallel techniques developed for *in vitro* fertilisation, embryo storage, and implantation, they allow great influence over the reproductive capabilities of domesticated animals.

As with micro-organisms, animals can be used to produce proteins. A gene for a particular protein, perhaps a vaccine, along with a promoter gene to ensure its expression only in mammary tissue, can be inserted into a sheep during its embryonic development. The sheep will then produce the protein in its milk from which it can be purified.[7] Already several useful compounds can be produced in this way using large farm animals, although none has as yet been produced commercially.[8] This technique may be more convenient for producing certain products, overcoming some of the disadvantages of culturing vast quantities of bacteria. Indeed, the opportunities are almost unlimited, by inserting the relevant genes into an animal, almost any imaginable protein of pharmaceutical or industrial interest could be produced in transgenic farm animals, we may even be able to produce complex structures, including essentially human organs for transplantation.

As well as using animals as producers of useful proteins, genetic modification also allows certain characteristics to be programmed into the animals themselves. Harvard University, in collaboration with Du Pont, has used genetic modification techniques to develop a mouse with an unusually high predisposition to cancer. These animals are designed to develop a breast cancer similar to that in humans; they can thus be used as a model for research into human disease. Research workers can use these 'oncomice' to study the molecular biology of cancer, and they are useful for assessing new treatments before they are tried in humans. Similarly, it is possible to develop mice with a predisposition to other cancers, and other diseases can be studied in this way.

The possible adverse effects of these genetic modifications are hard to estimate. Animals are more easily controlled than micro-organisms and so the fate of any novel genes introduced into a population should be more easily determined. Also, new genes can be introduced into animals in such a way that they cannot be passed to the next generation. Only a small number of the cell population of an animal is usually involved in reproduction, these being termed 'germ' cells, in contrast to the normal body

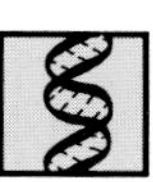

or 'somatic' cells. As many of the genetic modifications are likely to require changes only to somatic cells they will not be inherited by any offspring of the modified animal. This does, however, require accurate targeting of the novel genes, and in some instances the aim may be that a novel gene should be inherited, or as part of its function must affect germ cells.

Genetic modification in humans

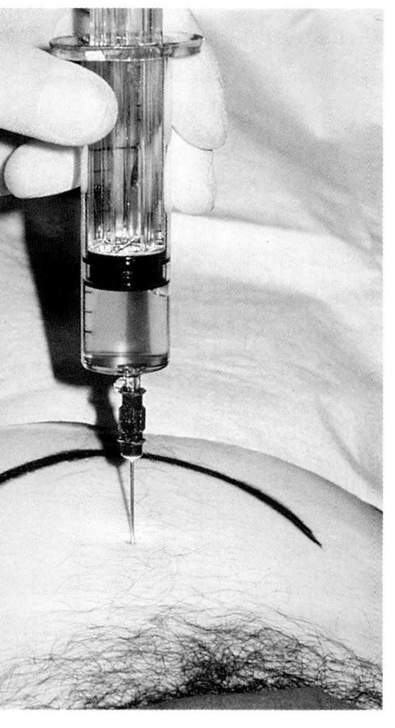

Amniocentesis: amniotic fluid is taken through a needle and then the DNA it provides is analysed to identify any genetic abnormalities in the foetus

One application of human genetic modification relies on the use of these techniques to identify abnormalities of genes associated with particular diseases. We can extract cells from a human foetus at a relatively early stage in its development by either amniocentesis or chorionic villus sampling. Specific segments of genes can be recognised, and if these foetal cells are found to contain an abnormal gene, the prospective parents may wish to request that the pregnancy be terminated. This technique could be helpful in identifying several inherited diseases, such as cystic fibrosis, or diseases such as sickle cell anaemia and thalassaemia characterised by abnormal haemoglobin (haemoglobinopathies), the pigment which carries oxygen in our blood. The World Health Organisation estimates that by the year 2000 approximately 7% of the world's population may be affected by these haemoglobinopathies, making them serious causes of morbidity and mortality.[9] Usually, only a proportion of the children of a couple who may be carriers of the defective gene will be affected, and so with prenatal screening couples who wished to do so could ensure that their offspring would not be affected. *In vitro* fertilisation techniques mean that doctors should be able to identify and implant only embryos without the defective gene, thus avoiding the need for termination.

Gene modification offers great potential benefits to man in the treatment of serious disease, so called 'gene therapy'. As our ability to alter genes increases we should be able to identify individual genes or groups of genes which are abnormal. These can then either be replaced by excising the incorrect gene and inserting a correct version, by correcting the genetic code contained in the abnormal gene, or by inserting a whole new functional gene to act in place of the abnormal gene without replacing it. Several diseases, such as cystic fibrosis, are caused by specific abnormalities in genes which theoretically we should be able to correct. Some other diseases have similar genetic causes, including sickle cell anaemia, the thalassaemias (one of the haemoglobinopathies mentioned above), forms of muscular dystrophy, phenylketonuria and other inborn errors of metabolism, to mention but a few. Genes are important, too, in that they determine at least, in part, some of the most common diseases including thyroid dysfunction, diabetes, and asthma, all of which are to some extent genetically as well as environmentally influenced. Our genetic makeup is also responsible for the body's ability to recognise its own cells and what is foreign material through the proteins produced on a cell's surface (antigens). Our own body cells can be recognised from these antigens, while mounting a vigorous response against cells bearing foreign antigens. Although generally important in

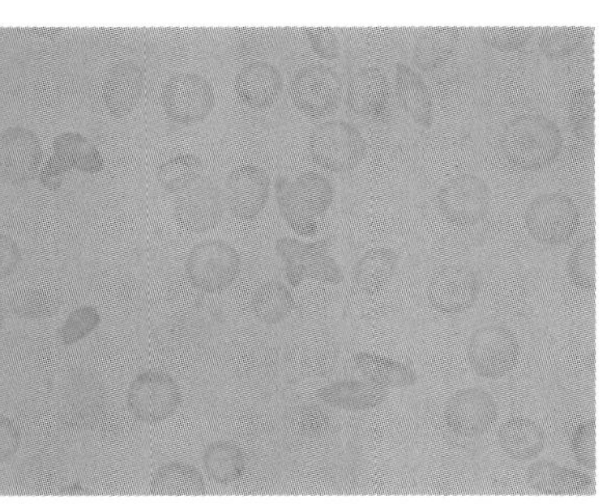

Sickle cell anaemia showing the characteristically sickle-shaped red blood cells

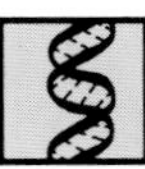

fighting infection, this self recognition facility has caused problems in transplant surgery, where organ rejection and failure have been common complications. The ability to manipulate the surface antigens on an organ to be used for transplantation would end the problem of rejection and the recipient's lifelong dependence on immunosuppressant drugs.

Somatic cell gene therapy, the correction of defective genes in particular tissues of the body, affects only the individual concerned and therefore is no different in principle from other routine and widely accepted therapies. As such, somatic cell gene therapy raises no new ethical issues but as with all innovative therapies it should be subject to rigorous ethical appraisal and used only when there is no alternative available or when it offers genuine advantages, such as safety or efficacy, over other types of treatment. With these reservations, somatic cell gene therapy has considerable potential.

Germ-line gene therapy, on the other hand, involves modifying genes in the reproductive cells which would cause changes not only to the genetic make-up of individuals but also to their descendants. At present the risks associated with germ-line gene therapy, such as genetic damage during the modification process or the loss of a gene with hidden advantages from the gene pool, are impossible to evaluate and there is a general consensus, that germ-line gene therapy should not yet be attempted. In the UK it is currently prohibited under the Human Fertilisation and Embryology Act (1990).[10]

Several occupational health risks will also become apparent to people working with these techniques, although relatively little has been published on these so far. As with any other laboratory work, they involve the exposure of staff to chemicals and other hazards, to which must be added the risk of exposure to genetic material, small amounts of which may have significant consequences. (See box on page 108)

Environmental effects of gene modification

Any estimate of the environmental impact of the applications of genetic modification to humans would be guesswork because so little is known about it. Gene therapy in humans is in its infancy. Ideally, any use of genetic material in humans should be thoroughly researched and strictly controlled. If this can be achieved, widespread adverse environmental effects seem unlikely but not impossible.

Regulations and guidelines

The high profile and emotive nature of gene manipulation have inevitably prompted public and professional anxieties about its possible consequences for our health and environment. Regulations to control the safety of genetic modification have been in place since 1978.[11] Specific regulations were introduced in 1989,[12] as well as parts of other more general legislation, to impose certain duties and responsibilities on companies, academic and

 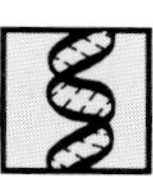

research institutions, or other agencies taking part in genetic modification or using organisms which have been so altered.[13] They are already required to notify the Health and Safety Executive of the details of their work, and to have made a full risk assessment of the hazards of their work. Despite these requirements it was felt that the 1989 regulations did not provide the same degree of protection for the environment as they did for human health and safety. Separate provision for the protection of the environment was also necessary in view of the likely increase in proposals to release genetically modified organising to the environment. Specific regulations for environmental safety were therefore introduced in 1992.[14] The Genetic Modification Regulations (1989) were replaced with the Genetically Modified Organisms (Health and Safety) Regulations (1992), to be broadly compatible with these environmental requirements.

Under the Genetically Modified Organisms (Contained Use) Regulations (1993) the Health and Safety Executive (HSE) must be notified of any level 2 work and what precautions are being taken. In February 1994 inspectors from the Health and Safety Executive halted research at a UK university when arrangements to contain a adenovirus, genetically modified to insert oncogenes into human cells, were thought to be inadequate. Although the chances of an accident were extremely small there was concern that the genetically modified virus could have triggered cancer if it had infected laboratory workers or the public.[15] Working with the Advisory Committee on Genetic Modifications the HSE has produced guidance on assessing the risk of particular types of experiments.[16]

The Committee on the Ethics of Gene Therapy (Clothier Committee) was succeeded by the Gene Therapy Advisory Committee in February 1993. The committee works closely with other agencies which have responsibilities in the field of gene therapy, including local research ethical committees, Medicines Control Agency, Health and Safety Executive and the Department of the Environment, to provide advice on the acceptability of proposals for gene therapy research on human subjects, on ethical grounds.[17] In the area of gene therapy there must be constant re-evaluation of the issues involved. Without such continuing re-evaluation there is a risk that decisions will be based merely on past accepted practice or on an intuitive distaste for certain proposals. Intuition has its place but must always be congruent with ethical and scientific reasoning.[18]

Work on plant pests requires, in addition, a licence from the Ministry of Agriculture Food and Fisheries, or in Scotland from the Department of Agriculture and Fisheries for Scotland. Any person or group wishing to introduce a product of genetic modification to the environment must also provide full details of the nature, size and purpose of the release, along with a full assessment of the environmental consequences. This assessment should include information on the likely survival and persistence of the novel organism, its ability to transfer genetic material, and methods to eliminate the organism. A contingency plan in the event of unplanned effects is also required. Responsibilities and duties as regards the occupational hazards of genetic modification are contained in current legislation including the Health and Safety at Work etc Act (1974), the COSHH Regulations (1988); and the Management of Health and Safety at Work Regulations (1993). A full assessment of the occupational risks of any work process should be carried out, including contingencies for emergencies and unforeseen circumstances. Health surveillance of employees is also required if the risk to health cannot be eliminated.

Discussion

The techniques of genetic modification have the potential through application in agriculture, medicine and technology, to increase the well-being of people and to promote the health of the population by disease prevention. Wrongly used, they also have the potential to cause harm. Those developing the techniques and applications of this new technology must consider the consequences of their activities. Existing regulations regarding genetic modification must be effectively enforced. In order to ensure the safety of workers in the field of genetic modification. National guidelines on training for work with bio-hazards, genetically modified organisms and other potential threats to the individual or to the environment should be established. At this stage in the development and application of genetic modification it is not possible to provide any guarantees against, or insurance for mistakes. When we seek to optimise the benefits over risks, it is therefore prudent to err on the side of caution and above all to learn from our accumulating experience.

Balance to be struck

A difficult balance has to be struck in regulating genetic modification to allow legitimate and potentially beneficial research to continue while protecting the community from possibly adverse effects on individuals and the environment.

CHAPTER 9

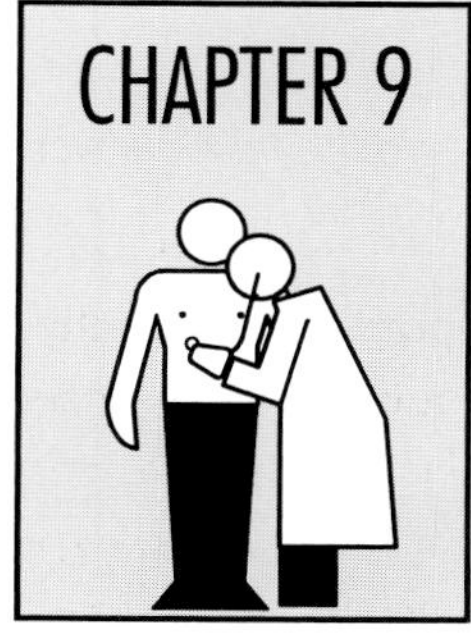

Occupational and public health

All doctors should understand how the environment may cause specific illnesses in their patients. Occupational and public health physicians, however, have a specific role in that part of their work is centred on protecting individuals from adverse effects of the environment. These two specialties often have a low public profile, since they spend less time in contact with patients than many other clinicians. Additionally, their colleagues in other medical specialties and the public may not always have a clear understanding of their role.

Occupational physicians are primarily concerned with the protection of the population from potential hazards arising at work. They may be responsible for, amongst other duties:

- Prevention and early detection of occupational disease
- Assessment of hazard & risk in the workplace
- Health surveillance
- Assessment of fitness to work
- Rehabilitation and return to work after illness
- Health promotion and education in the workplace
- Epidemiological studies of working populations

They assume responsibility for environmental health issues within and around the workplaces with which they are concerned. They have considerable experience in controlling exposure of the staff to potentially hazardous substances and physical agents in bulk, and in high concentrations, or in large-scale processes in which they are produced or used. This expertise may be extended in relation to the wider environment.

In the UK, the deployment of occupational health physicians should be a formal 'arrangement' to implement the statutory health and safety policy statement prepared and published by the organisation of which they are a part. Their primary role is determined by health and safety legislation, and must take account of the formal risk assessment which every employer is required to carry out.

Public health physicians employed by health authorities have a number of responsibilities, for example:

- Advise on the use of resources to provide the best service to a district population
- Act as officer and/or medical advisor to local authorities, especially environmental health departments
- Control of communicable disease — notification, surveillance and outbreak management
- Participate in the preparation of policies to improve the population's health
- Contribute to the management of health services in a health district
- Organise epidemiological studies of the population for which they are responsible
- Advise on problems of waste discharges from factories
- Advise on environmental monitoring

Governmental agencies

The Employment Medical Advisory Service (EMAS) was established in 1973, and subsumed within the Health and Safety Executive the following year, but outside of this, occupational health services in the United Kingdom have no formal regional structure. In addition to occupational physicians employed in EMAS organisations in the public and private sector have several large employed occupational physicians so that they have immediate access to appropriate advice. Some occupational physicians work in academic institutes within universities, whilst other doctors who are not fully qualified occupational physicians, mostly general practitioners, provide occupational health advice and services for smaller companies. Occupational health nurses and safety practitioners also make a valuable contribution to occupational health services. However, the lack of formal regional structure has led to services being distributed unevenly, so that less than 15% of all companies have access to occupational health services. Many firms see occupational health as an expensive overhead which is not essential, until something goes wrong, or the enforcing authority draws attention to failure to satisfy statute.

Doctors and nurses of HSE's Employment Medical Advisory Service have played a central role in the development of occupational health in the UK.

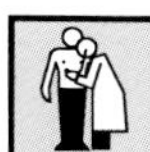

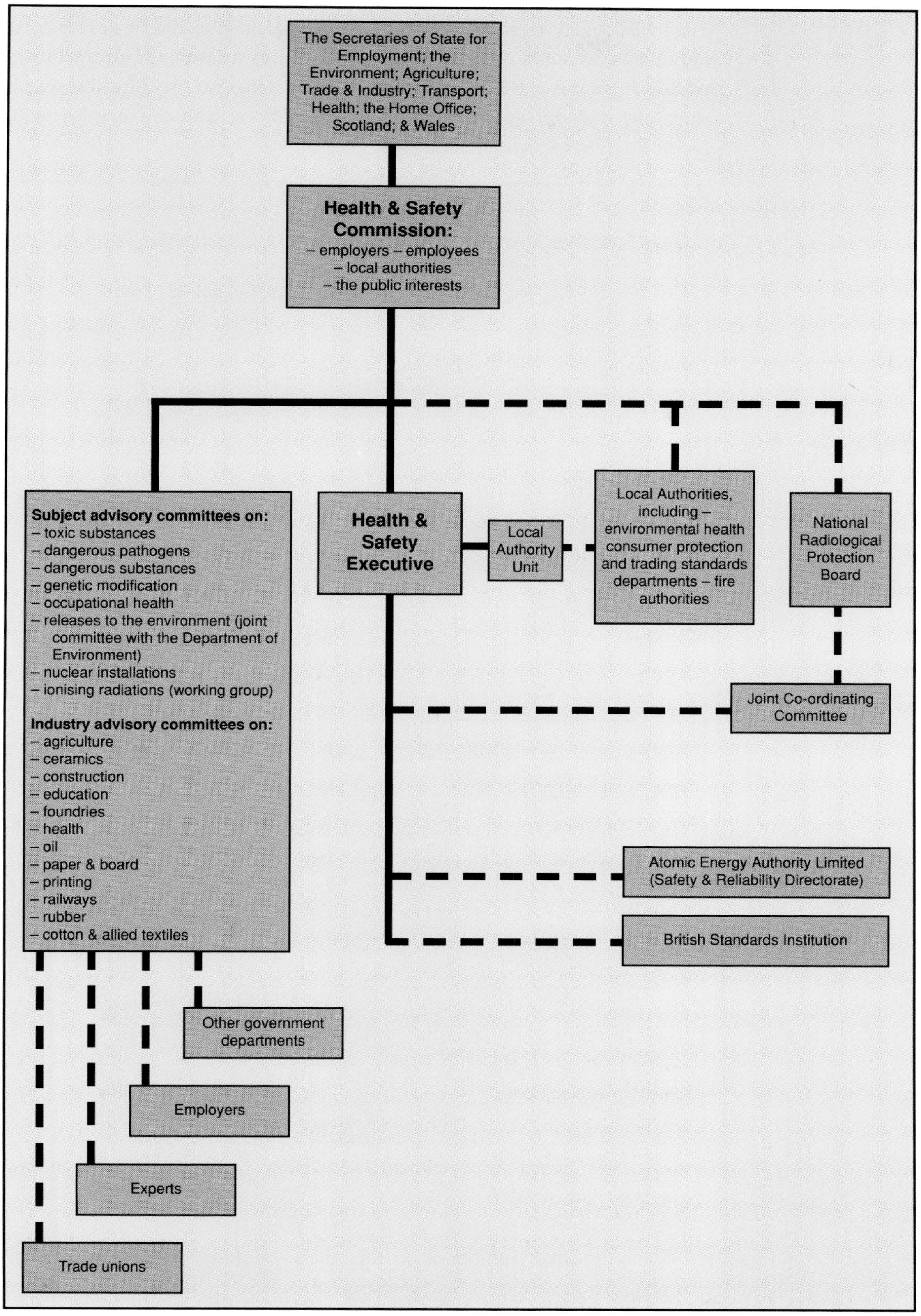

The Secretaries of State for Employment; the Environment; Agriculture; Trade & Industry; Transport; Health; the Home Office; Scotland; & Wales

Health & Safety Commission:
– employers – employees
– local authorities
– the public interests

Subject advisory committees on:
– toxic substances
– dangerous pathogens
– dangerous substances
– genetic modification
– occupational health
– releases to the environment (joint committee with the Department of Environment)
– nuclear installations
– ionising radiations (working group)

Industry advisory committees on:
– agriculture
– ceramics
– construction
– education
– foundries
– health
– oil
– paper & board
– printing
– railways
– rubber
– cotton & allied textiles

Health & Safety Executive

Local Authority Unit

Local Authorities, including – environmental health consumer protection and trading standards departments – fire authorities

National Radiological Protection Board

Joint Co-ordinating Committee

Atomic Energy Authority Limited (Safety & Reliability Directorate)

British Standards Institution

Other government departments

Employers

Experts

Trade unions

Figure 9.1
Health and safety institutions in Great Britain

They will usually seek to work by providing information and by persuasion, rather than by coercion. Unfortunately, some firms are deterred from seeking advice from these HSE medical and nursing advisors, fearing that legal sanctions may be applied to ensure compliance with the employment medical advisors recommendations.

Table 9.1
Days lost due to work-related illness by occupational group (UK)

	Illness caused by work	
Occupational category	*Days lost (000s)*	*Days lost/worker*
Professional	143	0.08
Teaching	287	0.33
Nursing	366	0.61
Other education	147	0.18
Literary, artistic and sports	60	0.16
Science and engineering	154	0.15
Managerial	314	0.13
Clerical	308	0.07
Selling	124	0.08
Security	184	0.39
Catering, cleaning and hairdressing	621	0.21
Farming, fishing and forestry	141	0.26
Processing (other)	510	0.33
Processing (metal and electrical)	730	0.32
Painting	72	0.29
Repetitive assembly, inspection	208	0.30
Construction	326	0.40
Coal mining	31	0.66
Transport and materials moving	452	0.31
Others (miscellaneous)	6	0.04
All occupations	5,184	0.21

Source: OHR Dossier. Accidents cost UK £16 billion. Occupational Health Review 1994, May/June. P19-21

Given the small number of doctors, nurses and inspectors employed by the HSE, the likelihood of a visit to one of over 900,000 small businesses is remote, so despite statutory powers of entry, their influence is limited. It is of great concern that the Government plan to reduce expenditure on the HSC by £5 million in 1994-1995 and £10 million in 1995-1996, with a cash

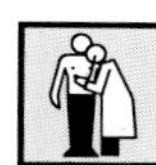

freeze thereafter.[1] Further resources are required by the HSC if it is to fulfil its role in protecting both employees and the public from the hazards of work processes, and if the improvements seen since the introduction of the Health and Safety at Work etc Act (1974) are to be maintained and furthered. The National Audit Office expressed concern about staffing imbalance between HSE Area Offices which may prevent inspectors in understaffed areas from carrying out time consuming work. eg prosecutions.[2] A case could be made that the cost of more HSE staff would be repaid many times over in the improved health and safety of workers. The costs of failing to manage health and safety successfully in the workplace are high. It is estimated that 30 million working days are lost every year due to work-related injuries and ill health and over the past decade there has been a two-thirds increase in real terms, of employers' liability insurance costs.[3] Dealing with accidents involving chemicals and biological materials is costly in time and money and human suffering.

Occupational health services were not included within the NHS at its inception in 1948, and subsequently their development within the NHS has been haphazard in comparison with public health, which itself has suffered from several reorganisations, during the past 20 years. Employees in the NHS have until recently been sadly neglected and occupational health services in hospitals are provided often in only a very rudimentary form. Even where occupational health services have been established, the main objectives are seldom understood by hospital staff. Only a few consultant occupational physicians have regional responsibilities for advising districts other than their own, and the numbers of consultant occupational physicians in the NHS is likely to be grossly inadequate for the 1.3 million NHS staff. The NHS requires a comprehensive consultant-led occupational health service to meet the needs of all staff including general medical and dental practitioners and their practice staff. Indifference in the NHS Executive contrasts starkly with the concerns of others involved in the health sector, such as large pharmaceutical companies, which as the norm rather than the exception, provide occupational health services.

As a result of pressure from the BMA, the NHS has been appointing a number of well qualified and experienced full time consultant occupational physicians who have by their own efforts established quality services. This has significantly improved the provision of occupational health advice to workers and the management of NHS hospitals. Regrettably some hospitals still have inadequate occupational health services, this is in any case short-sighted, a false economy and a disservice to staff. Furthermore, it fails to address the risks identified by fulfilling the statutory requirements of the Management of Health and Safety at Work Regulations (1992). These deficiencies should be remedied, as soon as possible, to ensure a national network of occupational physicians so that all health care workers and contractors in the private and public sectors have access to occupational health services. This provision should be a pre-requisite for approval of trust status, and access to the service should be required by all private hospitals.

Based on central guidance from the National Health Service Executive (NHSE) a coherent approach to the risks of health care must be developed across each region, and in each Trust. Each region should provide detailed guidance and advice to districts on the development and coordination of services. In the market-based NHS this is a service which could also attract valuable revenue by providing an affordable service to small employers. In the longer term, preventive medicine could lessen the pressure on NHS resources. However, to compete successfully with other occupational health services, such as those already formed by groups of employers, the NHS occupational health service will have to demonstrate that its practitioners are highly trained and well resourced.

Legal responsibilities

Health and safety in the workplace and the environmental consequences of an organisation's activities are governed by extensive UK and EC legislation. Occupational health services work within this framework, with a primary professional responsibility to eliminate or reduce work-related ill health in employees. They do this by advising employers and employees about potential hazards at, or arising from work. As companies' responsibilities for emissions, effluents and waste disposal extend beyond the place of work, so occupational physicians have expanded their responsibilities to giving advice about protecting the environment. The training of occupational health staff includes the legislation for attaining a safe and healthy environment. This encompasses domestic (UK) legislation, such as the Health & Safety at Work etc Act (1974) (HASAW), the Environmental Protection Act (1990), and the numerous regulations, codes of practice and guidance notes which stem from that Act and relevant European Community Regulations. Staff must be aware of international agencies and conventions such as the World Health Organisation (WHO), the International Labour Organisation (ILO), and their publications on occupational health and safety.

Legal responsibility for compliance with all relevant legislation in the UK rests corporately with the employer and specifically with the management. Since Crown immunity from prosecution was removed from the NHS, the HSE now has right of entry onto NHS premises to discharge its statutory responsibility including the provision of advice to management and the full enforcement of health and safety legislation. Managers in health service units may be prosecuted by the Health and Safety Executive and fined individually or even imprisoned for gross failure to comply with the minimum standards. The HSE, can be expected to serve Improvement or Prohibition Notices on recalcitrant employers, to enforce measures to improve an unsatisfactory environment or to ensure that authorities, trusts, or general practices exercise their general duty of care. Women at work should be protected routinely from physical, chemical, biological and psychological risks to health, but during pregnancy, the control of hazards is particularly important. Pregnant women should be protected from specific hazards which may damage the

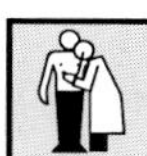

foetus, or, if this is impossible or impractical, temporarily redeployed. Since women make up approximately 70% of the NHS workforce, this is not an insignificant issue. UK legislation already exists to protect staff from these dangers, and further legislation is being drafted from an EC directive aimed at protecting pregnant workers and those who have recently given birth.[4]

The Health and Safety at Work etc Act (1974) covers the environment in and outside the workplace, if it affects the health or safety of contractors or visitors (including patients) and the general public. In addition, the Environmental Protection Act (1990), which can be similarly enforced by HM Inspectorate of Pollution (HMIP) the Waste Regulation Authorities and local authorities, regulates disposal of waste and emissions from factories and other undertakings. The Government is in the process of bringing together all the functions of the HMIP, Waste Regulation Authorities and the National Rivers Authority to form a new Environment Agency. This legal framework applies to NHS hospitals, research establishments, private hospitals, independent contractors such as general practitioners and to the pharmaceutical and medical engineering industry.

Stress at work

Environmental factors play an important part in the production of stress. For example, the working environment will be a determining factor in levels of occupational stress. Examples of such occupational stressors for medical staff include the risk of occupationally acquired infection and exposure to hazardous substances. In addition to specific hazards in the workplace, doctors' workload may also be harmful. Junior doctors suffer some of the longest hours of work and most arduous training of any employed group, and from a relatively young and inexperienced age they may face high levels of responsibility and the stress of making difficult decisions. Even when fully trained, many doctors continue to work well over 40 hours a week; much of this work will be difficult, requiring both prolonged spells of concentration and often responsibility for making life and death decisions.

The interface between professional life and community life is particularly stressful for general practitioners. As they work from home and work unsociable hours, it is impossible for family doctors not to involve their

Stress and general practitioners

Stress is also a problem for general practitioners. A study by Makin et al[5] isolated four major sources of stress:

- interruptions,
- emotional involvement,
- administrative workload and work/home interface,
- routine medical work.

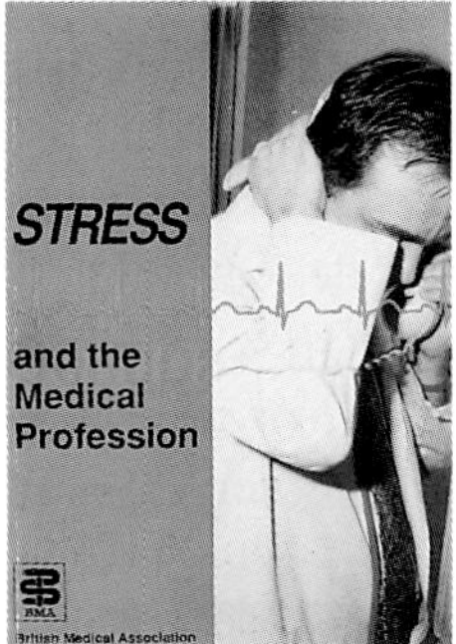

families in their work, particularly due to the 24 hour continuing commitment to patients.

Many within the medical profession are concerned that the burdens of long hours, of difficult and stressful work, must have consequences upon health. Furthermore, although some aspects of a doctors' work are potentially harmful, they are an inescapable part of the job. The BMA's comprehensive report *Stress and the Medical Profession,*[6] published in 1992, showed that stress is an urgent problem within the medical profession itself, evidenced by the high rate of suicide, alcoholism and drug abuse found in doctors. The study confirmed that stressors faced by health professionals not only affect their own health, but may adversely affect patient care and the health service as a whole.

The occupational physician's responsibilities for assessing fitness to work, rehabilitation and health promotion and education in the workplace means that they have an important role in identifying stress in individual doctors and in the management of the adverse health effects of stress in the medical profession.

It is also important to deal with environmental factors. If stress is dealt with on a purely individual basis, the individual may find their personal symptoms dealt with, only to be returned to the environment that led to stress in the first place, even though they may be more able to cope. Occupational physicians can also play an important part in putting pressure on management for changes in the working environment where unacceptable levels of ill health due to stress can be identified. Improvements in occupational health facilities for health workers would undoubtedly make an important contribution to identifying and controlling stress-related illness within the medical profession.

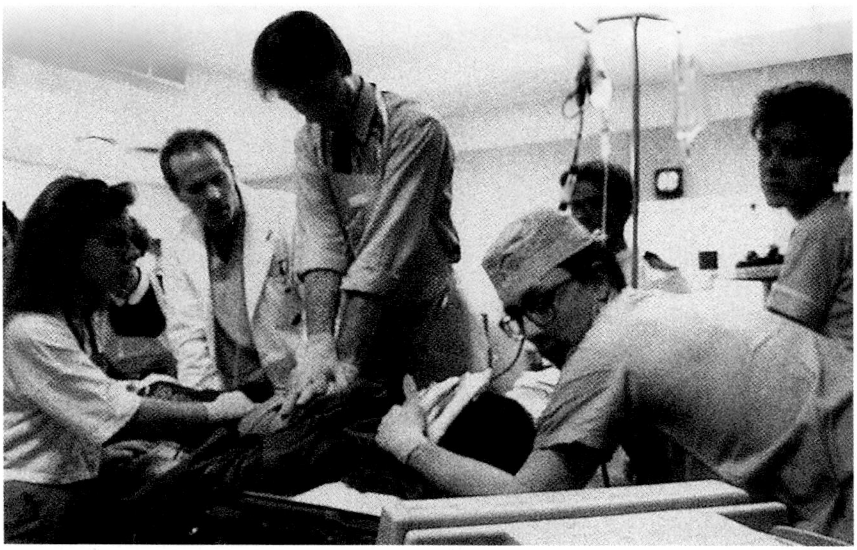

From a relatively young age junior doctors face high levels of responsibility and the stress of making difficult decisions

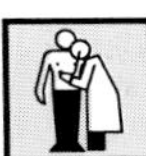

LABORATORY PRODUCTS: MATERIAL SAFETY DATA SHEET

FORMALDEHYDE & RELATED MATERIALS

CHEMICAL SYNONYMS	FORMULAE
Formaldehyde	HCHO
Methanal, formalin	
Hexamine	$(CH_2)_6N_4$
Hexamethylenetetramine	
Paraformaldehyde $(HCHO)_3$	Poly Methanal

GENERAL: These materials liberate formaldehyde gas under various conditions. Formaldehyde gas is widely used as a disinfectant and germicide and these materials have been used medicinally.

Formaldehyde solution is a solution of formaldehyde gas in water which contains approximately 12% methanol. It is used also in the manufacture of several organic chemicals including artificial silks, the production of mirrors, tanning and in photography.

TOXICOLOGY: Toxic, irritant or harmful by ingestion, inhalation or skin contact.

Formaldehyde is a protoplasmic poison but is primarily irritant in action. The gas has a strong irritant effect and a concentration of 100ppm will give rise to severe toxic effect and definite irritation of the eyes and upper respiratory tract. Symptoms of poisoning by ingestion include; Gastro-intestinal upsets which are painful and frequent, blood stained vomiting, suppressed urine, vertigo, depression and coma.

Formaldehyde gas is more toxic than formaldehyde solution, hexamine and paraformaldehyde. The control exposure limit for formaldehyde vapour is 2ppm, 2.5mg/m3.

HANDLING PRECAUTIONS: Workers handling formaldehyde solution should follow the advice on the EEC Hazard Labels. In addition, we would recommend for all materials the following precautions:-

Laboratory: It is preferable to use formaldehyde in a fume cupboard and any work that requires heating of formaldehyde, hexamine or paraformaldehyde should always be carried out in a fume cupboard. Normal laboratory protective clothing and effective eye protection should otherwise prove suitable.

ACCIDENT ACTION:

a) Skin Contact: Remove any contaminated clothing and wash the affected area with water, then soap and water. If exposure has been prolonged or severe seek medical aid.

b) Eye (s): Irrigate the affected eye with cold running water and obtain immediate medical assistance.

c) Ingestion: Obtain immediate medical assistance.

d) Inhalation: (Of formaldehyde vapours) remove the individual to fresh air, loosen any constricting clothing and make him lie flat. Obtain immediate medical assistance.

(of solid dust) - blow nose and clean nostrils with moist cotton wool. If soreness or irritation persists seek medical assistance.

Figure 9.2: Material safety data sheet

occupational hygienist, who is trained to assess and measure exposure using recognised scientific techniques. Judgement on the risks of exposure to hazardous agents in the workplace requires skill in interpreting toxicological and epidemiological data. Whilst occupational physicians receive some training in toxicology and epidemiology they may not have specialist expertise in human toxicology. They are unlikely to have comprehensive knowledge about the effects of all agents on all biological systems, since the range of information is enormous. Occupational and public health physicians should be trained in and be familiar with all the steps for investigation of occupational and environmental health (see box on page 122), so as to identify cause (exposure) and effect when health problems arise. The specialties of occupational and public health medicine emphasise complementary skills in identifying and controlling environmental hazards both inside and outside the workplace. Thus co-operation between the two groups of physicians is essential if environmental problems in the NHS are to be tackled successfully.[12]

The Faculty of Occupational Medicine has found that 88% of the 570 members and Fellows regarded environmental medicine as an integral part of occupational medicine and were already practising it, and 80% regarded a change of the Faculty's title to incorporate environmental medicine as being appropriate. Occupational medicine specialists increasingly find themselves advising on the potential or actual health impacts on the public of workplace through their operations and their products. This report has shown that the NHS workplace can present risks to the wider environment and hence to the general public. A clearly defined extension of the role of the occupational health doctor, to cover all the risks that the workplace may present to health, both within and outside the working environment, would seem appropriate. The Faculties of Occupational Medicine (FOM) and of Public Health Medicine (FPHM) of the Royal College of Physicians — the professional bodies responsible for education and qualifications in the two specialties — have already established a joint committee to advance the role of medicine in environmental issues among both specialties. Expert advice on occupational health matters can, of course, be obtained from the Medical Division of HSE and they should be consulted in the early stages of planning safe working places and practices as well as about the monitoring of existing working environments.

Any health care employee who believes that his or her work is being affected by the workplace environment should have ready access to occupational health staff. The same facility should be available if staff believe the environment is being adversely affected by working practices. Detailed reporting of all accidents, ill health and dangerous occurrences should be routine practice and satisfy the requirements of The Reporting of Injuries, Diseases and Dangerous Occurrences Regulations (1985) (RIDDOR). Subsequent analysis of the records produced will provide data for epidemiological studies into possible environmental effects on the health of staff and patients in the health sector.

With the HSE, the NHS Research and Development Directorate should review the need for research into occupational and environmental problems in health care and consider this issue as a priority area for funding. The Occupational Health Advisory Committee and Health Services Advisory Committees of the HSC and HSE should assist individual occupational health departments to act as sources of advice upon the need for research into existing and newly emerging occupational and environmental problems in the NHS. A central database of research in this area should be established through the NHS Research and Development Directorate with the results widely disseminated throughout the health service. The central database would then enable the NHS to issue guidance to local units based on currently available research evidence. Employers would also be able to consult the database to gain access to information on current research into occupational and environmental health in the NHS.

Occupational hygiene

Occupational hygiene is a related but separate discipline to occupational health. Hygienists do not normally have medical training but their skills

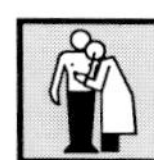

include the careful and systematic investigation and evaluation of any possible environmental hazards. Private consultancy firms and academic departments staffed by skilled occupational hygienists are a good source of occupational hygiene advice and service. Nevertheless, occupational physicians and nurses should be able to recognise and make a preliminary analysis of the environmental hazards associated with simple problems such as noise and toxic gases, etc. Inexpensive instruments are available to measure sound and radiation levels and concentrations of toxic gases in the environment. Only trained staff should operate and interpret results, otherwise the readings may give a false sense of security or provoke undue alarm.

Once an occupational hygiene survey has been done and areas of concern defined, appropriately trained occupational physicians and nurses should be able to monitor the environment regularly. The three main elements of occupational hygiene, clinical assessment and epidemiological analysis enable the occupational health service to advise managers on the dangers to the environment of advances in health care. They should be widely applied in the health sector.

Education and training of occupational and public health specialists

The Faculty of Occupational Medicine (FOM) of the Royal College of Physicians, London was founded in 1978 to establish standards of knowledge and competence in occupational medicine. It arranges a series of examinations, firstly, for the Associateship of the Faculty (AFOM), which is a written, oral and practical examination, secondly, for the Membership of the Faculty (MFOM), which is awarded following a presentation of a satisfactory dissertation. Finally the Fellowship (FFOM) is awarded to members of distinction and those who have contributed to the Faculty or the specialty of occupational medicine by election from amongst the established members. In 1994, a Diploma in Occupational Medicine will be introduced which will be available to medical practitioners, with a limited or part-time interest in the practice of occupational medicine. They will follow a Faculty approved training course and take a Faculty examination.

Training in public health medicine involves at least 7 years at general professional, basic specialist and higher specialist levels. Doctors enter at registrar level and progress to senior registrar posts. An academic course is followed which may also include a masters degree (MSc or MPH) and leads to Membership of the Faculty of Public Health Medicine (MFPHM) Part 1. Part 2 is awarded following presentation of a satisfactory dissertation and *viva voce* examination covering general aspects of public health medicine practice. On entry to the specialty many doctors already have other clinical qualifications. Subjects covered during training include epidemiology and statistics, communicable disease, environmental health and health service planning and evaluation.

Nurses have for many years taken additional qualifications in occupational health. The qualification of Occupational Health Nursing

Certificate (OHNC) is awarded by the English National Board for Nursing, Midwifery and Health Visiting after a period of training and a written and practical examination. The Royal College of Nursing awards a BSc in Health Studies (Occupational Health) which includes a set number of modules in occupational health.

The British Occupational Hygiene Society, is a learned society and does not award qualifications or accreditation, although it facilitates continuing professional development. The British Examining Board in Occupational Hygiene (BEBOH) governs written Preliminary Certificate examinations and Certificate and Diploma level examinations comprising both written and oral elements. Professional accreditation is awarded by the Institute of Occupational Hygienists (IOH) who consider practical experience and academic record based on either the BEBOH preliminary cert/certificate/diploma, or acceptable equivalents together with the relevant BEBOH or IOH oral examination.

A Health and Safety Executive lead body is currently defining the role and responsibility of the occupational physician, the occupational nurse, the occupational hygienist and the safety officer who are the multi-disciplinary team responsible for the delivery of occupational health.[13]

Continuing education

It is important to recognise the importance of continuing education in all specialities related to environmental and occupational medicine. The FOM, like its parent body the Royal College of Physicians, has recently appointed a continuing medical education liaison officer who will carry forward progress in continuing medical education for all occupational physicians. As in many other branches of medicine scientific advances continue at a fast pace. In occupational medicine there is also the continuing march of legislation, both within the United Kingdom and within the European Community as well as guidance issued by bodies such as International Labour Organisation and the World Health Organisation. Occupational health practitioners must keep up to date with all these advances and be fully aware of the employers' responsibility, as well as that of the employee, in the prevention and control of occupational hazards.

CHAPTER 10

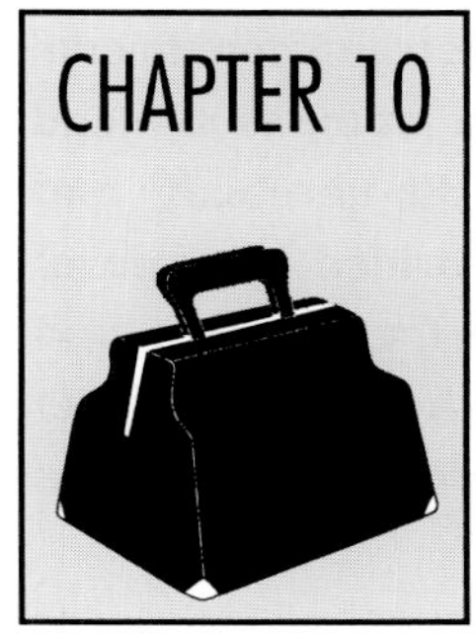

General practice: health, safety & environmental issues

The general practitioner (GP) is not an employee of the health service, but an independent contractor and as such, has a different relationship with the NHS to that of doctors working in hospitals. This is an important difference which shapes and directs the way in which general practice is managed and develops. As an employer, the GP assumes a number of important responsibilities affecting the general practice environment and the health and safety of his employees, and anyone else who enters the premises. This chapter therefore, discusses some matters which appear elsewhere in this report, such as health and safety legislation, clinical waste and infection control, but in the context of the particular needs of general practice.

The structure of general practice

During the past forty years of the National Health Service general medical practice has greatly expanded and consolidated its role in providing first line health care services to the population. The number of GPs has increased from about 18,000 in 1949 to well over 32,000 in 1994, and are supported by a further 2,700 GP trainees and assistants. The average number of patients on each GP list is approximately 2,000 and each patient makes about 4 visits to the GP per annum. More than 80% of general practitioners are in partnerships whereas at the outset of the NHS the single handed practitioner was in the majority. The physical structure of general practice has changed to accommodate group practitioners, allowing a great expansion of practice staff from a few hundred at the beginning of the service to in excess of 40,000 whole time equivalents in 1990. A 1993 national census of practice nurses indicates that there are about 16,000 nurses employed by GPs and this number is likely to increase.[1]

Responsibilities of the general practitioner

The GP has a contract to supply services to patients on his list, who are registered by the Family Health Services Authority (FHSA). It is his responsibility to provide the premises, time, equipment and systems to do an appropriate job. There is considerable flexibility about how and where this service is provided within the broad guidelines of the contract. The contract between the general practitioner and the FHSA contains agreements about hours of work, access by patients, and standards of premises. General practitioners are required to, "render his patients all necessary and appropriate personal services of the type usually provided by general practitioners" and, "shall keep adequate records of the illnesses and treatment of his patients on forms supplied to him for the purpose by the authority" and, "shall do so at his premises or if the condition of the patient so requires elsewhere in his practice area".

The FHSA has the responsibility of planning, developing and managing services provided by general medical practitioners, general dental practitioners, retail pharmacists and opticians. The role of the FHSAs includes supporting continuing education for the staff in practices, encouraging medical audit as well as traditional tasks such as inspecting premises, approving surgery locations and hours of availability.

Managing the new NHS[2] proposes important changes in the central management structure of the NHS to streamline administration and consolidate joint working between DHAs and FHSAs. The 14 statutory Regional Health Authorities (RHAs) will be abolished and the National Health Service Executive will be reorganised, to include 8 regional offices. DHAs and FHSAs will be enabled to merge to create stronger local purchasers. Such changes are planned to support the continued drive towards decentralisation in the NHS, with responsibility and decision making devolved as far as possible to local level.

Health and safety in general practice surgeries

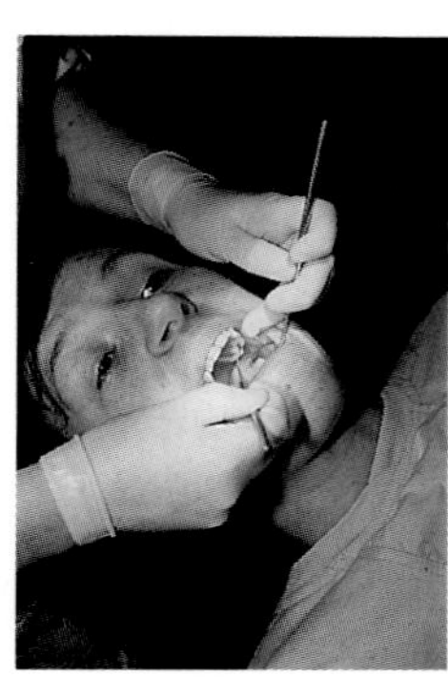

Family Health Service Authorities has responsibility for general dental as well as medical services

Surgery premises are included in the 'health services' grouping and they are subject to the Health and Safety at Work etc Act (1974), and inspection by officials of the Health and Safety Executive (HSE), who may visit GP surgeries from time to time to ensure that the general practitioners are maintaining a healthy and safe working environment.

The main aim of the Health and Safety at Work etc Act (1974), is to ensure that both the employers and the employees must do all that is reasonably practicable to ensure a safe working environment. The general practitioner must ensure that particular hazards or risk of injury have been assessed and action taken to reduce the risk of injury as far as possible. The Act requires equipment and methods of working to be safe and not to pose a risk to health. There are many physical and electrical hazards in a general practice environment such as word processing equipment, photocopy machines,

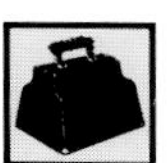

(1990) a duty of care has now been placed on those dealing with controlled waste. The duty requires those responsible for controlled waste to take all reasonable measures to:

- prevent it causing environmental pollution or harm to human health
- ensure that it does not escape from their control (eg by packaging it securely)
- ensure that it is handled only by someone authorised to receive it (eg a registered waste carrier or disposal licence holder); and
- to ensure that, when waste is transferred, a transfer note, sufficiently describing the waste, is handed to the recipient.[5]

This duty does not apply to occupiers of domestic property as regards their household waste.

All general practitioner surgeries should have an infection control policy which is understood by all employees and which details the procedure to follow in the event that a member of staff or a general practitioner experiences a needlestick injury or blood exposure. The British Medical Association has produced codes of practice to help general practitioners to establish their own practice policies.[6,7]

Physical hazards

In the expansion of computer technology in the workplace, general practice has been no exception. The Display Screen Equipment Regulations (1992) which came into force on the 1 January 1993, places specific duties on employers with regard to VDU users. Staff who use VDU equipment need to avoid eye strain and have comfortable seating and be able to adjust the brightness and contrast of the screen image. Staff will require to take short but frequent breaks away from the visual display unit (VDU) equipment. Employees who are covered by the regulations can ask for an eyetest.

The Manual Handling Operations Regulations (1992) require that employers should identify all manual handling operations undertaken by employees and seek to enable them to avoid risk of injury where possible, and provide training and instruction, to enable them to undertake necessary handling in safety. The use of mechanical aids, eg a sack truck or trolley, should be considered when reasonably practicable to improve safety and also productivity.

Implementation of the Provision and Use of Work Equipment Regulations (1992) applies to all sectors of work activity where any machine, apparatus, tool or installation used at work is involved. The employer must ensure that work equipment is suitable, without risks to health or safety and is adequately maintained. Control systems must be safe and breakdown or damage must not result in danger.

There must be protection against rupture or disintegration of equipment and there are further requirements for any electrical equipment. The Electricity at Work Regulations (1989) state that all electrical equipment in the workplace must be constructed and maintained to prevent danger so far as is reasonably practicable. Portable appliances must be tested by a certified competent person who is capable of using the 'testing' equipment. This does not need to be an electrician, however, all repairs must be carried out by a qualified and registered electrician. Staff must know how to operate electrical equipment safely and may require special training. Trailing wires on the floor or from desks must be avoided to prevent physical injury.

Employees' responsibilities

Employees are required to take reasonable care for their own health and safety on the premises and for the safety of other users of the premises who may be affected by their actions, throughout the time that they remain on the premises. This would include the full working day as accidents can occur in the staff room or whilst preparing refreshments in a kitchen. Staff must not interfere with or misuse any equipment provided for health and safety purposes, ensure that fire exits are not blocked and know where fire extinguishers are located.

Occupational health services

Legal responsibility for compliance with all relevant legislation in the UK rests with the employer (including independent contractors such as GPs). Like all other employers in the UK, they have moral and legal responsibilities to ensure that all their staff receive adequate training in how to prevent accidents and occupational diseases. GPs may make special arrangements with the local NHS consultant in occupational health for advice and guidance on health and safety of themselves and their staff.

Enforcement

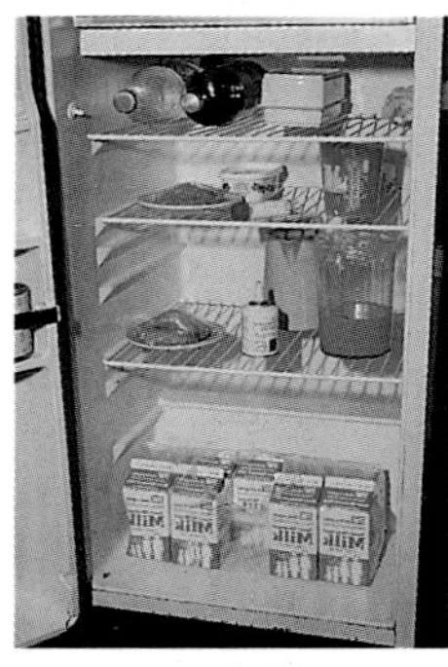

Pharmaceuticals and chemicals must be stored safely away from food

Failure to carry out any duty under the Health and Safety at Work etc Act (1974), and the COSHH Regulations not only exposes people to unnecessary risk, but constitutes an offence and can lead to prosecution. The Health and Safety Executive is firstly an advisory body, and has the discretion to decide when prosecutions are required. The courts would then assess what is reasonably practicable in the light of considerations such as available resources. An inspector would normally give prior notice before arranging a visit to a general practice and very rarely are inspections made without discussion, in response to a complaint from an employee or user of the premises. Inspections will cover a wide range of matters within the practice, covering electrical equipment, toilet and washing facilities, heating systems, arrangements for sterilising instruments, disposing of clinical waste and safe storage of drugs.

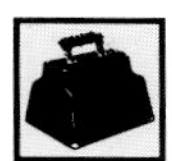

General medical practice premises

Grants may be available to fund improvements to general practice premises, or new premises if the FHSA's prior approval has been obtained. As with many other businesses, there is a number of reasons why a general practitioner may decide that his present premises are unsuitable. These may include their size — either too large to heat or ventilate adequately; too small for current services or storage needs; or unable to accommodate a planned expansion of services or staff numbers. An expiring lease, for instance, may necessitate the practice finding new premises. It is important for general practitioners to contact the FHSA and its medical advisor at an early stage when planning substantial alterations or new premises, and in assessing options for design. The FHSA will, however, have to take account of its predetermined priorities and its cash allocation when considering an application. Advice on the standards of accommodation is given in paragraph 56, Schedule 1 of the 'Red Book'.[8] The briefing and design principles for general practice premises are provided in Health Building Note 46 *General Medical Practice Premises* published by the NHS Estates Agency,[9] whose services are described in more detail in chapter 11.

Alterations to existing buildings or the building of new premises should take account of health and safety aspects and security aspects of general practice. Wide doorways, grab rails and avoidance of steps are beneficial not only to those in wheelchairs but also to parents with small children, the elderly or the infirm and to a certain extent other users of the building. GPs and practice nurses should be provided with good treatment room facilities with appropriate privacy, space for preparing instruments, testing specimens and storage of equipment, and with sufficient space for the nurse's clerical duties and computer equipment. All practices need a secure space for the storage of medicines and this is particularly important in dispensing practices. All controlled drugs must be kept in a locked receptacle.

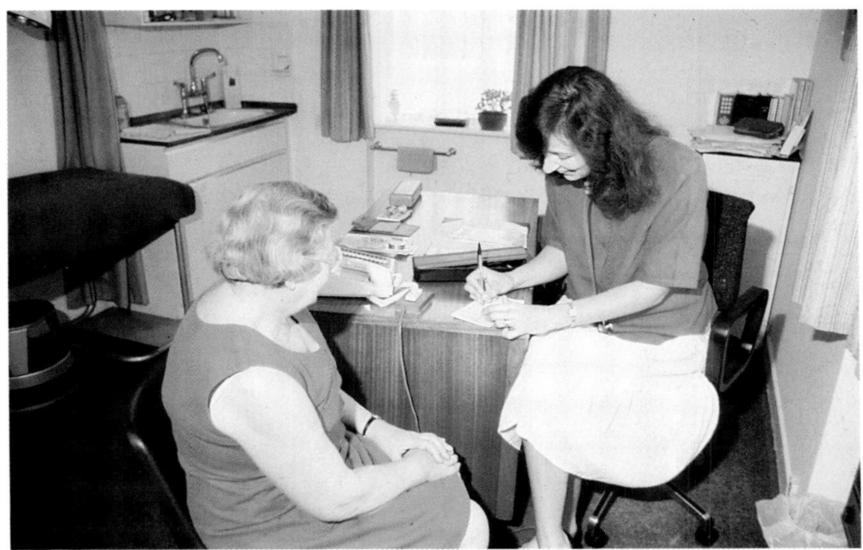

GPs and practice nurses should be provided with good treatment room facilities with appropriate privacy

Discussion

General practitioners have an important role to play in identifying occupationally-related morbidity and mortality as they will attend to the health problems of a far greater section of the community then occupational health doctors. General practitioners are encouraged to discuss confidentially, suspected occupational illness or injury with the relevant occupational health department, to gain appropriate advice and to assist in the maintenance of occupational health records. General practitioners also have a vital role in identifying morbidity and mortality that could be related to environmental factors. The detailed recording of information and collation of results by general practitioners and occupational health doctors is necessary in order to identify preventable deaths and illness, and enable proper assessment of the impact of medical technology and health care processes on patients, staff and the environment.

Environmental and occupational health concerns are likely to proliferate as a result of the changes now taking place in general practice. Increased health screening services, further delegation of duties to practice nurses, and the expansion of community care are extending GP responsibilities, and must be managed with care to avoid causing additional health problems. Clinical waste generated in the community will need to be safely disposed of to prevent infection and should be reviewed in conjunction with local FHSA's. The delegation of certain procedures further intensifies the need for practices to provide appropriate staff training. Infection control policies with adequate follow-up procedures, in the event of sharps injury or blood exposure must be introduced.

Guidelines on good practice and infection control should be the standards used in an audit process to ensure continuous quality improvement. It is only by reviewing practice in infection control that the risk of infections can be reduced and quality of care improved. Monitoring the effectiveness of infection control programmes is a way of measuring outcomes and therefore reflects the quality of care given to patients.

CHAPTER 11

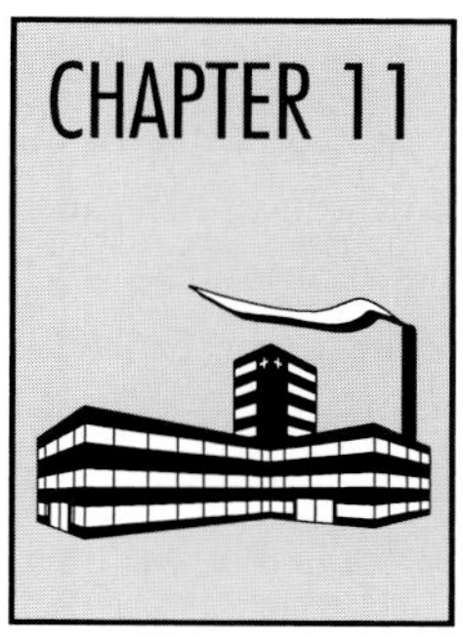

Building design and environmental management

The NHS estate is one of the largest landholdings in England. It costs over £3 billion a year to run, including capital charges, and investment in new buildings is now approaching £1.5 billion a year. Effective design and maintenance of this complex and important resource can improve the quality of health care and reduce the hazards associated with the use of medical technology.

The design of buildings for 'specialist' use is based on expert knowledge and experience and those in the health sector are no exception. Architects and planners have to take account of many factors, including ventilation, lighting, waste disposal, gas and electricity supply, access, siting of laboratory or x-ray services, position of water towers, and many other features. Badly designed structures may present a hazard to health or necessitate time-consuming maintenance and repair, which interrupt normal activities and disrupt the care of patients. Designs which enhance patient care, safeguard the health of staff, and have minimal impact on the environment are self-evidently of benefit to the community.

NHS buildings have been funded by the Department of Health's capital programmes. Comprehensive guidance on design and construction is provided by the NHS Estates (an Executive Agency of the Department of Health) in the form of Health Building Notes and Technical Memoranda which cover building design and engineering technology relating to new and existing premises. The Health Building Notes are based on research and consultation with health care staff, and provide insights into the planning and functional content of entire buildings or departments. The standing of these notes is enhanced by the Treasury's acceptance of their cost effectiveness. The Health Technical Memoranda detail more specific aspects of building services systems for health care. These include such diverse factors as medical gas pipeline systems, nurse-call systems, sterilisers, and special ventilation systems for operating theatres. They cover the design, operation and continuing safety aspects of building systems operation and are based on research and extensive consultation with the various groups concerned in planning and using buildings.

Nucleus design system

'Nucleus' is a comprehensive design system offering a briefing and planning concept for a complete hospital or hospital department. It incorporates proper standards of clinical care and service with maximum economy in capital and running costs. Its use is specifically supported and recommended by the National Audit Office, the Parliamentary Accounts Committee and the NHS Executive. There are approximately 140 major schemes in the NHS drawing on 'Nucleus'. Most importantly use of 'Nucleus' can overcome the problem of shortages of skilled planning and design staff in both health authorities and the private sector. This and other information is available to outside organisations, such as private hospitals.

Much recent legislation on building design has been centred on protecting employees health, but other legislation is also relevant to building design.[1-5] Certain aspects are covered by codes of practice or guidelines, such as the report of the Advisory Committee on Dangerous Pathogens.[6] The official framework for building design is completed by various British Standards. In addition several professional bodies provide a range of advice on building matters.

Hierarchy of risk assessment

Parliament has incorporated the principles of risk assessment and control in much recent legislation directly or indirectly affecting the health sector. In 1993 the then NHS Management Executive published a comprehensive guide to risk management in the NHS.[7] This acknowledged the important role of risk management in ensuring a high quality, safe service for patients, as well as protecting staff and the environment. A risk assessment must be undertaken for any hazard in the workplace. If a significant risk exists it should be reduced. The COSHH Regulations list a hierarchy for reducing risks from hazardous substances. This includes:

- Elimination or substitution of the hazardous substance
- Control of exposure by controlling access to the substance if elimination or substitution is not possible
- Enclosing the process
- Provision of appropriate extraction or dilution ventilation.

Most chemical and microbiological hazards can be controlled if risk assessment and control is applied following these principles. Although most legislation covering safety in the workplace does not apply to patients being treated, it does cover visitors to a hospital or clinic, including

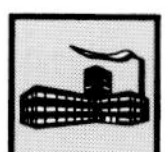

medical/nursing/health service students etc, and it also applies to patients in respect of substances being used in their treatment.

The hazards of health care in so far as they influence building design can be grouped under three headings:

- chemical hazards
- infectious hazards
- general environmental considerations — heating, ventilation, lighting, etc.

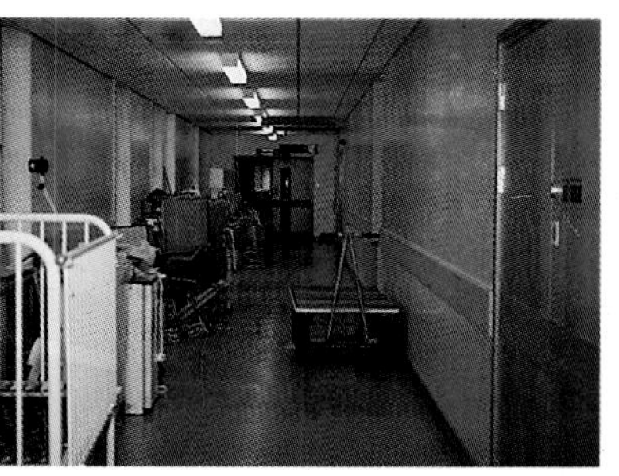

'Sick building syndrome' has been associated with artificial ventilation and lighting

This classification encapsulates such diverse issues as exposures to specific chemicals within laboratories, to general comfort and, of more recent concern, the sick building syndrome — a disorder associated with artificial ventilation and lighting causing a distressing group of symptoms, including headache and nausea. Many of these issues are not specific to health care, although there may be special requirements to be considered in this setting. Hospitals have many areas necessitating special precaution for cleanliness, and several chemical substances and pathogenic micro-organisms may exist in the health sector which are not widely encountered elsewhere.

Chemical hazards

Examples of potentially hazardous chemicals are glutaraldehyde and formaldehyde, used as disinfectants, fixatives, and preservatives; anaesthetic gases; cytotoxic drugs used in treating cancer; and methyl methacrylate, used as a bone cement in orthopaedic and dental surgery. The hazards they present have been discussed in earlier chapters, and in this chapter we focus on how building design and improvements in the workplace can reduce or eliminate the risks to patients, staff and visitors.

The rapid expansion of day surgery and, particularly, endoscopy has brought with it a major chemical exposure hazard. Fibreoptic endoscopes, with their delicate optical systems, cannot be disinfected by autoclaving. This has led to the increasing use of glutaraldehyde for disinfection, which is active against a wide range of infectious organisms including mycobacteria and HIV. This chemical may be dangerous to staff using it due to the likelihood of sensitivity reactions. The techniques used for chemical disinfection with glutaraldehyde range from semi-automated processes, to crude manual manipulation in containers. Both processes — particularly the latter — can lead to staff being exposed to the chemical and appropriate exhaust ventilation is required, preferably close to where the endoscopes are used. To reduce the exposure of staff, disinfection should ideally be done in an isolated part of the endoscopy unit, preferably in a dedicated disinfection room or zone. Even something as simple as disposal of empty glutaraldehyde containers should be planned because seemingly trivial exposures can cause symptoms. Disposal areas should therefore have adequate ventilation and be sited away from areas where unintended exposure may occur.

Glutaraldehyde is contained in chemicals used for the processing of x-rays but adequate planning should ensure integration of film processing equipment with exhaust ventilation devices so as to prevent staff being exposed. Unfortunately, sporadic cases of skin and respiratory sensitisation continue to occur among radiology staff.[8] The recent development of digital imaging, processing, and transmission of diagnostic data means that traditional film technology may eventually become obsolescent, thus removing this exposure risk.

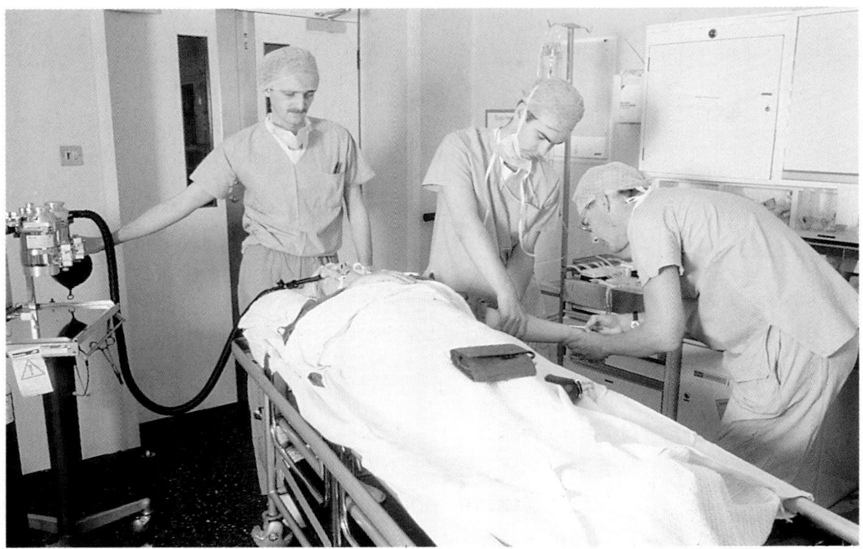

British Standard Specifications set safety criteria for anaesthetic gas scavenging systems

The administration of anaesthetic gases to patients in operating theatres are covered by a British Standard Specification that gives criteria for anaesthetic gas-scavenging systems[9] and the NHS Estates Agency guidance which suggests that mechanical ventilation systems are sufficient to maintain an air change rate of 15 theatre volumes per hour.[10] The combination of these two measures is usually adequate to ensure a 'safe' exposure of staff. Even so, circumstances occur where the direct connection of a breathing system to a scavenging device is difficult if not impossible. Examples are dental surgery, maternity delivery suites and postoperative recovery areas. Despite this, good design of the working environment can at least help to reduce the hazards. Research in dental surgery by the NHS Estates Agency has shown that a combination of local exhaust, built into dental chair headrests, and nasal mask scavenging, can cut levels of exposure to those encountered in modern operating theatres. Such systems are not, however, widely used. The design of delivery suites in maternity units should include adequate scavenging systems.

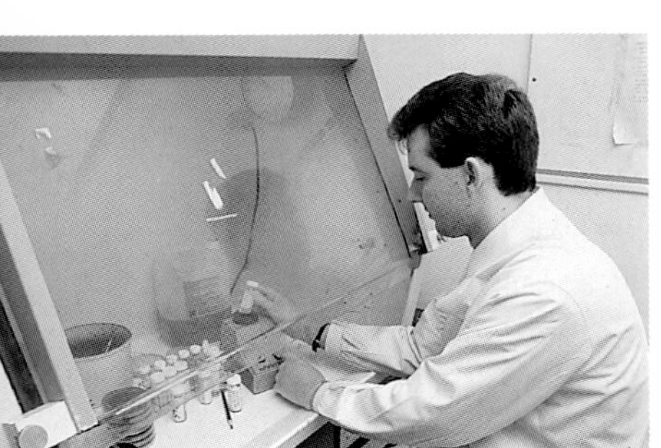

Exhaust protective devices require significant 'make-up' air to replace the large volumes of air extracted

One difficulty in providing a safe building environment is the extent to which the various safety features incorporated are mutually compatible. Virtually all exhaust protective devices require significant "make-up air", to replace the large volumes of air extracted. Such replacement generally has

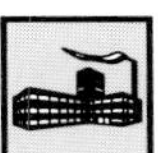

to be heated to maintain a comfortable working environment. This can be accommodated within a new building design, but is not always easy to provide in an existing building. Fume cupboards with an integral make-up air supply which does not require heating have been developed. However, the British Standard on Class II Safety Cabinets (which are classified as competent for the manipulation of cytotoxic agents) shows that there is uncertainty about the performance of such devices, especially those requiring a large volume of air for containment and dilution.[11] The development of absorption-filtration for recirculating fume cupboards may be helpful in the control of certain agents. The main problem, however, is one of regular maintenance to ensure that the absorptive matrix is checked for saturation and replaced when necessary. However, these devices have yet to show that their aerodynamic performance provides adequate containment of hazardous gases. Nevertheless, they do provide one way of redeveloping existing facilities to provide a safe environment.

Infectious hazards

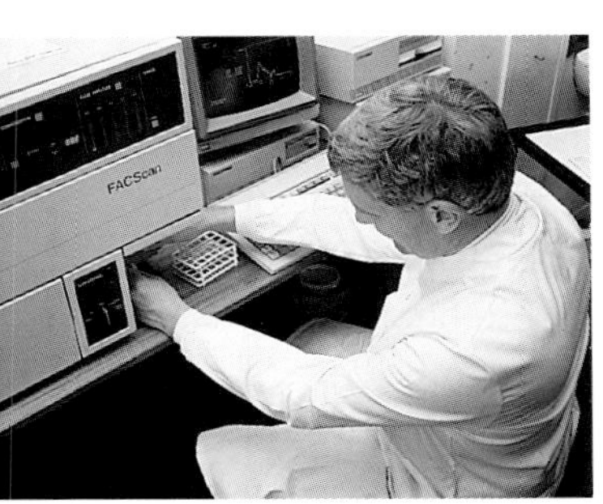

Routine haematology may bring the health care worker into contact with pathogens

Infection may originate from patients, visitors, staff, laboratory areas, clinical and non-clinical waste, and the buildings in which the services are provided. Prevention of spread of infection in health care facilities is covered by the COSHH Regulations. Specific advice for laboratories is available from the Advisory Committee on Dangerous Pathogens[12] who recommend precautions to ensure safety appropriate to the pathogenicity of the micro-organism in question, and the processes being undertaken. Simple benchwork with a normally non-pathogenic micro-organism requires fairly simple safety precautions. By contrast, work with the most pathogenic micro-organisms is subject to several requirements. Micro-organisms are categorised into four hazard groups that correspond to an equivalent numerical level of containment. For work where it is known what pathogens are being used, the numerically corresponding containment levels directly apply. However, in diagnostic laboratories there will be uncertainties about the presence of pathogens in the materials being handled and containment levels will need to reflect the likelihood of pathogens being present.

The emergence of new infectious diseases has prompted a wide ranging review of the provisions in health buildings. These have to be flexible to cover those suffering from HIV to the more intractable problems of multiresistant strains of airborne organisms. A Department of Health working party is reviewing the need for such provisions and the protection and/or isolation required when handling various micro-organisms. Health building guidance has to encompass a range of criteria from staff facilities to maintain simple clinical hygiene — for example hand washing — to the elaborate control of air flow within such accommodation and the provision of air locks.

Control of airborne spread of disease is a fairly well established practice and few problems should occur if up to date structural technologies and ventilation systems are used to ensure an adequate level of security and containment. That said, good design alone is not sufficient. Sophisticated building services require continual monitoring and maintenance to ensure their long term reliability. No design, however good, can compensate for inadequate maintenance or failure of simple infection control techniques.

General environmental considerations

Hospitals and clinics, as is the case with other large workplaces, must provide a suitable environment for a variety of work. To achieve this many modern buildings require artificial ventilation because the size is often too large to allow effective natural ventilation. Furthermore, areas such as computer rooms or operating theatres usually have special requirements in respect of the temperature or humidity of incoming air. All this means that cooling, heating and humidifying equipment has to be an integral part of the design of modern health care facilities. Lighting, too, is important, since many areas in modern hospitals do not have any natural light.

The artificial environment of many modern workplaces, including hospitals, has resulted in those working in them developing the 'sick building syndrome', a disorder seemingly associated with artificial ventilation and lighting. Whether in the long term a specific cause for this distressing group of symptoms will be identified, which include headaches, nausea, inability to concentrate and lassitude, is unclear. Meanwhile it should be possible to design buildings so as to minimise its incidence and effects. A sensible provision is to plan natural ventilation and lighting where possible. If this cannot be done, staff should be provided with some control over their environment. Staff would also be helped if the flicker from strip lights was eliminated and the artificial lighting mimicked the colour spectrum of natural light.

Legionnaire's disease is another building-induced health hazard, cooling towers used for air conditioning plant, and hot and cold water systems have proved to be good culture mediums for *Legionella* bacteria. Effective water treatment regimes should eliminate the risk of infection from cooling tower water, but good design is also essential. Siting cooling towers away from air conditioning intakes is a sensible precaution but it has not always been adopted. Similarly, exhaust from any extract ventilation should be sited away from air intakes. Infection from hot and cold water service systems is harder to combat. Any agent added to curb micro-organisms must not detract from the potability of the water. The traditional assumption has been that water delivered to hospitals is wholesome and thereafter, the aim has been to prevent infection from *Legionella* and other micro-organisms. The design and maintenance of water systems should control temperatures and thus prevent colonisation and growth of pathogenic bacteria. This remains sound advice. On occasion, however, antibacterial agents may be added within the concentrations permitted for drinking water, to help where patients are at particular risk or where the quality of the installation is suspect. A Health Technical Memoranda exists for the control of *Legionella* in health care premises and provides recommendations, advice, and guidance on the

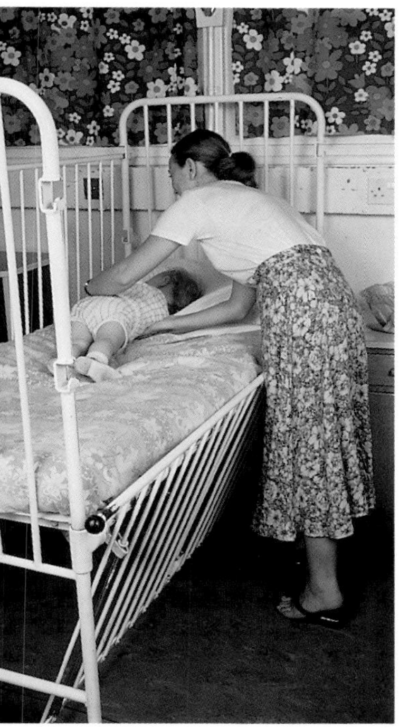

Wards should be laid out to enable lifting without contortion

control of *Legionella* in health care premises.[13] The guidance focuses on legal and mandatory responsibilities of estate and general managers and the design, maintenance and operation of systems. Further technical memoranda are planned for hot and cold water supply, storage and mains services and the ventilation of health care premises.[14]

Ergonomics and VDUs

Ergonomic factors may also contribute towards discomfort or ill health. Most importantly in the health service are the problems associated with patient lifting and handling. Back pain is one of the most serious occupational hazards in nursing. However, the difficulties resulting from the need to lift and manipulate patients could be partially resolved by appropriate ward design. Beds on which the height can be adjusted should be used as standard and layout of wards should be such that there is adequate room around beds, in toilets and bathrooms to enable lifting without contortion. In addition to the problems associated with lifting are the problems resulting from the poor design of office layout and furniture. Again back problems can result from inappropriate office design particularly in relation to the provision of appropriate chairs with adjustable height and back rests.

Visual display units (VDU) are widely used throughout the health service however, research has failed to identify any harmful effects of their use. Although difficulties may arise where VDU operators have inappropriate workstations in which to work comfortably there is a lack of evidence for harmful effects on vision or pregnant women. In relation to visual problems it is usually the case that the use of a VDU brings to light a pre-existing problem. Regulations exist in relation to manual handling and VDUs and the Health and Safety Executive has issued a guidance on these issues.[15,16]

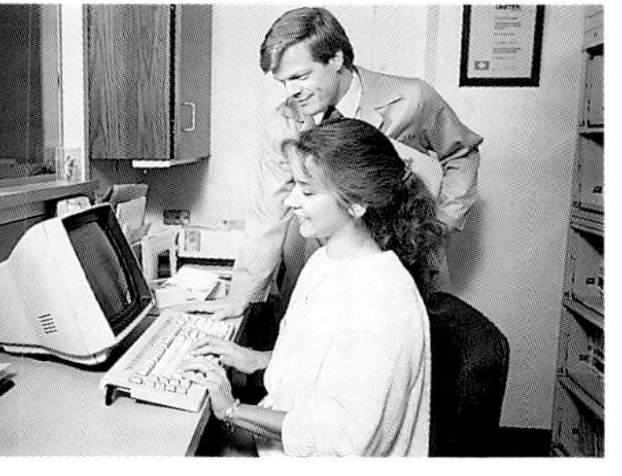

VDUs are widely used throughout the health service

Energy conservation

Another important aspect of environmental protection is the conservation of energy resources. There is a growing awareness of the need to reduce energy consumption and the harmful emissions produced by burning fossil fuels and to fulfil these aims the Government has outlined a strategy for sustainable development. This calls upon all sectors of society to participate in developing effective national strategies that meet present needs without compromising the well-being of future generations.[17] One of the targets set by the Government is to achieve an energy saving of 15% over five years for all government departments.[18] Energy consumption, and other areas of the Government's sustainable development strategy such as in development and construction, and waste disposal, should be taken into account by the NHS Estates Agency in providing guidance in the health service.

Flexibility in building design

The buildings and infrastructure in the health sector help to determine the quality of care. They may cause or prevent hazards, and good design is

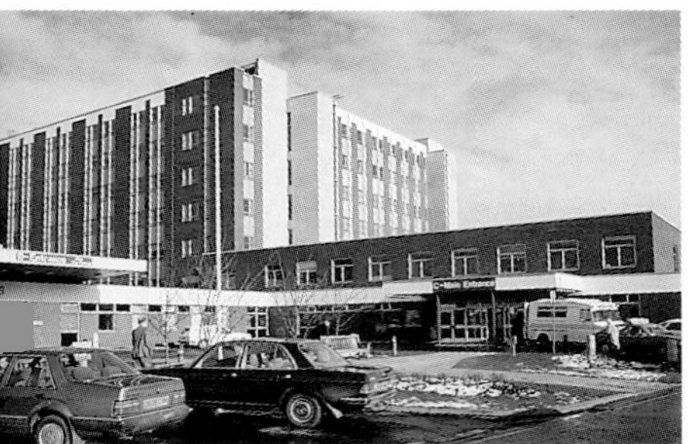

The buildings and infrastructure in the health sector help to determine the quality of care

central to the aim of controlling risks to staff, patients, and visitors, and to minimising the environmental impact of the health sector's activities; but quality costs money. Optimal designs for buildings and building services such as water supply, ventilation, and the disposal of waste are neither cheap nor easy to achieve. The pace of change within the health care sector compounds the problem. New treatments or techniques are being introduced all the time and hospital design, which is a long process, may inevitably lag behind medical advances. Many often conflicting criteria have to be accommodated. Flexibility in building design is therefore a high priority, so that future innovation can be incorporated in existing structures at minimum cost. Investment in design skills and planning is needed as well as in bricks and mortar. An indicator of the complexity of the task is evident from a recent report by the National Association of Health Authorities and Trusts. This authoritative body envisages a future in which a handful of high technology hospitals will serve the UK, with the majority of those patients who, in the 1990's, are treated as inpatients receiving their care in local communities, mostly on a day basis.[19]

Environmental management systems

Implementation of an environmental management system

The introduction of environmental management systems (EMS) is a fairly recent development in the UK. The British Standard BS 7750 (1993) and the EC's Eco-Management and Audit Regulation (1993) both provide a generic framework for the monitoring of environmental performance.

The British Standard BS 7750 specifies the elements of a general environmental management system which is intended to apply to all types and sizes of organisation, and lends itself to all aspects of the health care sector. A system of this kind enables an organisation to establish procedures to set an environmental policy and objectives, achieve compliance with them and demonstrate such compliance to others. The British Standard also compliments the draft European Community Eco-Management and Audit Regulation (1993). The draft regulation establishes a voluntary scheme, membership of which requires participating companies to have an internal environmental protection system.

The NHS, like all other major organisations is increasingly required to achieve and demonstrate sound and effective environmental performance. They must do so in the context of increasingly stringent legislation which is now in place within the health care sector to ensure that all hospitals, general practice surgeries and other health care settings are compliant in environmental matters. The proposed Environment Agency[20] will have a key role in the development of long term policy and in setting national standards in this area.

Consideration of the environmental factors associated with health care will be important in taking forward the Government's strategy on sustainable development which was one of the four main products of the UN

Conference on Environment and Development (Earth Summit) held in Rio de Janeiro in 1992.[21] In order to develop informed policy decisions the proper tools of analysis have to be applied to measure the benefits and damage to the environment associated with health care. Such tools include environmental management and schemes such as BS7750 and Eco-Management and Audit.

Environmental audit

Although environmental auditing is currently undertaken on a voluntary basis, it is an important development to help health providers to anticipate legal obligations and prepare for action. The Northern Regional Health Authority for example have piloted BS 7750, the British Standard which has been prepared under the direction of the Environment and Pollution Standards Policy Committee, in response to increasing concerns about environmental protection and environmental performance. The British Standard contains a specification for an environmental management system for ensuring and demonstrating compliance with stated environmental policies and objectives. It also provides guidance on the specification and its implementation within the overall management system of an organisation.

The Northern Regional Health Authority Health Care Pilot Study was based on a generic model of 12 very different pilot sites within the Northern Region, ranging from a large teaching district general hospital, a chemist shop; and an ambulance service — to a division of the NHS supplies authority.

The pilot study was structured to ensure that each of the organisations involved would receive some benefit. According to early reports of the study, one of the major advantages has been the links developed with suppliers, including the water industry, sterile dressing manufacturers, petroleum suppliers and the paper industry.

Objectives for environmental protection

The objectives for environmental protection should include a commitment to a continual improvement in overall environmental performance in a proportion of the areas of activity. (See box on page 146)

Targets for improvement should include those where they are most necessary to reduce risks to the environment and the organisation. Liabilities should be identified by cost benefit analysis where practicable. Targets derived from the objectives should be quantitative and achievable and may even involve components of personal accountability and performance appraisal for employees.

The work programme will include conducting preparatory environmental reviews and assessing the environmental effects of the pilot sites with the creation of a database and the development of appropriate performance indicators. The final study should aim to produce a manual

Seven key objectives for environmental protection

1. To minimise actions which directly or indirectly cause pollution of air or water from radiation, biological or chemical sources;
2. To minimise energy expenditure and maximise energy conservation in all activities;
3. To minimise the use of non-renewable resources, maximise the use of recyclable or renewable resources and maximise the recycling of all resources used;
4. To minimise actions which threaten plant or animal life and maximise efforts to conserve and promote wildlife habitats;
5. To maximise efforts to provide safe, aesthetically pleasing and health promoting indoor and outdoor built environments;
6. To minimise actions, economic and physical, which are detrimental to sustainable development in the UK or other countries of the world, and maximise efforts to promote sustainable development in the same;
7. To maximise efforts to promote environmental protection through education of public and professionals, active leadership, community development and collaboration with other organisations in all sectors.

and guidance notes particularly where training and performance appraisal of staff is involved.

The Royal College of Nursing has produced an environmental guide *50 Steps Towards A Healthy Environment*[22] which is designed to encourage nurses and other health professionals to take personal and professional responsibility for the environment in which they live and work. The guide also forms the basis for a simple audit tool to assess employers policies and strategies for dealing with the impact of health care activities on the environment.

Training for environmental management

All individuals within a health institution have environmental responsibilities and the EMS should be able to demonstrate that an effective training schedule is in place for all staff to develop their environmental competence. This should include health care practitioners as well as staff employed in hospital maintenance and service provision. The aim should be to raise staff awareness of the environmental impacts of their individual work and the environmental regulations associated with it. Occupational health departments have an important role in environmental management and are well placed to identify any risks from health care processes and technology

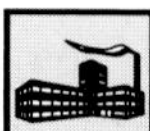

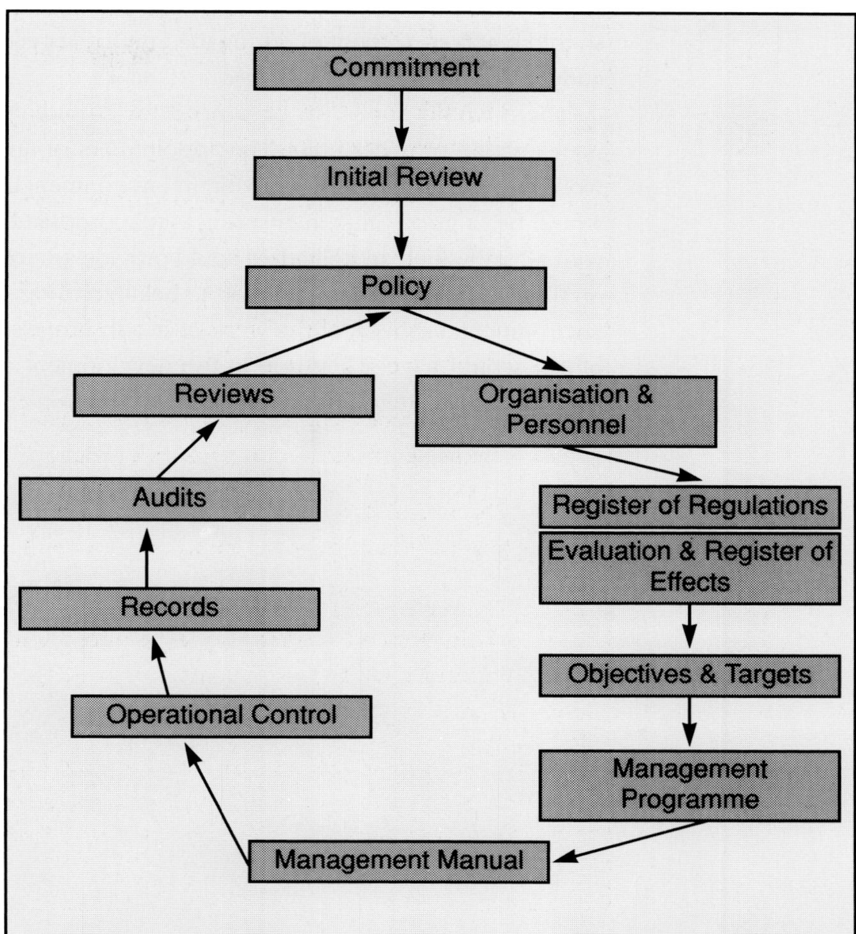

Figure 11.1: Environmental management system

on the environment and local population. In many industries this role has become well defined with occupational physicians being aware of the difficulties of removing hazards from the workplace to protect the workforce, whilst ensuring this does not entail their release into the wider environment with all the health risks this may bring. Occupational health staff within the NHS therefore need to be trained to provide advice on environmental management systems.

An opportunity to communicate and reinforce other health and safety legislation such as the COSHH Regulations (1988) and the Health and Safety at Work etc Act (1974) can usefully be undertaken during this training. Legal and financial consequences of poor work in practice should be explained and every effort made to improve communication on environmental issues which effect the organisation can be undertaken.

There is increasing awareness that health care providers in the service departments in hospitals should be provided with improved safety and environmental health training such as porters, nursing auxiliaries and other workers and it is likely that environmentally relevant duties such as the handling of clinical waste will be subject to improved training requirements, such as the General National Vocational Qualification (GNVQ) scheme. This should be taken account of during the training aspects of the environmental audit process.

There would appear to be a need for co-ordination of environmental issues within provider units. The appointment of an environmental officer would enable coherent local action in environmental risk management and would be of great value in ensuring that appropriate training is undertaken with all staff. Such an individual could provide advice to managers and staff on their responsibilities in relation to health and safety and co-ordinate the environmental aspects of the work of health professionals. In addition, the officer would have a key role in the development of local environmental management systems and in monitoring their implementation.

A strategy for control

The costs of failing to manage health and safety successfully in the workplace are high. It is estimated that 30 million work days are lost every year due to work related injuries and ill health and over the past decade there has been a two-thirds increase in real terms of employers' liability insurance costs.[1] Dealing with accidents involving chemicals and biological materials is costly in time and money and human suffering. Whether counted in human or financial terms, experience has shown that real and substantial improvements can be achieved by applying total quality management to health and safety. Each year in Europe and the USA, thousands of health care workers become infected with hepatitis B virus at work. Worldwide, 64 health care workers are known to have become infected with HIV at work, and a further 118 cases are presumed to have resulted from treating patients.[2] The first cases of patient-to-patient transmission of HIV[3] and possibly HCV,[4] have been reported from Australia.

The BMA's comprehensive report *Stress and the Medical Profession*[5] published in 1992 showed that there is an urgent problem within the medical profession itself, evidenced by the high rate of suicide, alcoholism and drug abuse found amongst some doctors. The study confirmed that the stressors faced by health professionals not only affect their own health but may adversely affect patient care and the health service as a whole. Long working hours, rapidly introduced NHS reforms, and the introduction of purchaser-provider contracts bringing the need to succeed in financial, as well as medical terms, have all produced new pressures and concerns for the profession, particularly in general practice.

The then NHS Management Executive recognised the importance of a healthy workforce by introducing a systematic healthy workplace programme in August 1992. In launching the action pack to help NHS workplaces become healthier, Sir Duncan Nichol, the then Chief Executive of the Executive, stated, "the Health at Work Initiative aims to make the

NHS an exemplary employer, demonstrating to others that a healthy workforce benefits both individual staff members and the organisation as a whole. This will help us to provide better services to patients. Healthy staff are in a better position to care for others".

Most of our medical technology and health care processes are relatively safe; problems may stem mainly from failure to manage health and safety policies effectively. Risks can be reduced but only by ensuring that procedures are correctly followed, that staff are properly trained and that the working environment is safe, and effectively managed. Reducing risks also requires managers to keep working hours and workloads within safe limits. Health care staff, their patients and the public will look to the responsible authorities to take action on the recommendations of this report in order that the risks of modern medical practice may be minimised.

Training for health and safety

Environmental pollution and environmental health as subject areas are being incorporated into the UK educational system as part of the schools' National Curriculum, the National Vocational Qualifications (NVQ) system of accreditation, and as undergraduate and postgraduate courses in higher educational establishments. There is a growing consensus that environmental and occupational issues should be addressed in the education of health care workers. All those employed in the NHS should enter with a basic knowledge of environmental health and safety, or receive such training upon commencing work. Effective training will help people to acquire the skills, knowledge and attitudes to make them competent in the health and safety aspects of their work, whatever their position in the NHS.

Induction and health and safety training at present are patchy and often inadequate. Many aspects of training in the NHS are likely to be based on 'on the job' observation rather than the use of clearly identified health and safety training programmes and protocols. A programme of training needs to take account of the individual job, the requirements of the organisation and its users, and the needs of the individual. Once these requirements have been identified, training objectives can be prioritised and used as a basis for auditing the training process. Training needs to be evaluated to ensure it is effective in developing a culture within the health services that gives a high priority to health and safety issues.

With many doctors now undertaking a managerial role, it is essential that they have an understanding of health and safety matters and their responsibilities in this area could be incorporated into doctors' contracts. Apart from health care workers, it is important that all those involved in the generation, handling, treatment and disposal of waste arising in the health service should also receive appropriate education and training.

Occupational health service

The low priority which has been given to occupational health services in the NHS is unacceptable. Even where occupational health services have been established, the main objectives are not always apparent to hospital staff. Only a few consultant occupational physicians have regional responsibilities for advising districts other than their own, and the numbers of consultant occupational physicians in the NHS may be grossly inadequate for the 1.3 million NHS staff. The NHS must establish a comprehensive consultant-led occupational health service to meet the needs of all staff including general medical and dental practitioners and their practice staff. To ensure that all health care workers have access to occupational health services, their provision should be a pre-requisite for approval of trust status, and should be required in all private hospitals. A coherent approach to the risks of health care must be developed across each region, based on central guidance from the National Health Service Executive (NHSE). Each NHS Region should provide guidance and advice to districts on the development and coordination of services. With the abolition of Regional Health Authorities in 1996 these responsibilities will need to be appropriately relocated.

Many of the problems identified in this report are unlikely to be satisfactorily resolved unless the recommended occupational health services are established throughout the NHS, to implement a national health and safety policy. The occupational health service should provide an extensive range of facilities to NHS employees and management, including health hazard evaluation; infection control services such as immunisation programmes for NHS employees; health promotion within the workplace; counselling and health assessments; and training and information, particularly in health and safety legislation and stress management. Public health input may drive this where NHS occupational health is not yet adequately established through the contracting process.

Health professionals are frequently called upon to work long hours and to make crucial decisions using sophisticated medical technology.[6] Any potential risk associated with such medical technology may be minimised or eliminated by the interventions of the occupational health service, to facilitate changes in working practices and environment, of mutual benefit to managers, employees and patients.

Contracts negotiated between industrial or commercial organisations often include requirements for health and safety provision for suppliers' staff and the public who will use the products. Purchasing authorities should follow this example and ensure that adequate levels of occupational health provision are maintained by the trusts or directly managed units, with which they are contracting.

Developing an environmental policy within the health services

The BMA report *Hazardous Waste and Human Health*[7] recommended the establishment of an Environmental Protection Executive (EPE). However, several years later the UK still lacks such a national agency to carry forward initiatives in environmental protection, and to oversee environmental health issues. In 1993 the Secretary of State for the Environment outlined the Government's plans to establish an Environment Agency for England and Wales by bringing together all the functions of the National Rivers Authority, Her Majesty's Inspectorate of Pollution and the waste regulation work of the local authorities. A similar organisation will also be set up to deal with Scotland.

A Bill has been introduced in the House of Commons to lay the foundations for the new Environment Agency, which should be operating in 1995. The Environment Agency will have a key role to play in combating pollution, with the following responsibilities:

- the power to assess the need for, and develop major long term policy on, all aspects of environmental protection and enhancement;
- set national standards of environmental and pollution control at least as high as those in the relevant EC Directives,
- be responsible for carrying out the existing (or proposed) pollution control functions for the Waste Regulation Authorities, Her Majesty's Inspectorate of Pollution and the National Rivers Authority, in discharge of which it would monitor the work and regularly assess the performance of pollution control officers working at local level.

In relation to the health care services, the Environment Agency could commission new research, oversee the regulatory framework and be responsible for drawing up national strategies and guidelines, eg for the disposal of clinical waste. The establishment of an Environment Agency would overcome many of the difficulties experienced in tackling environmental issues in the health care sector due to the current separation of environmental responsibilities between the Department of the Environment, the Department of Health, and the Health and Safety Commission. The Environment Agency should advise the Department of Health, the NHS Executive and the Health and Safety Commission and ensure that they comply with the national environmental strategy. The composition and powers of the Environment Agency will need to be considered carefully, to ensure its authority and independence. (Figure 12.1)

Within the industrial sector, companies are increasingly paying attention to the environmental effects of their technology and processes. However, changes to NHS management proposed in *Managing the New NHS*[8] fail to address the environmental health issue. Given the potential adverse effects of health care technology and processes on the environment, outlined in this report, the NHS Executive should dispatch its managerial responsibilities, in developing an environmental policy for the NHS.

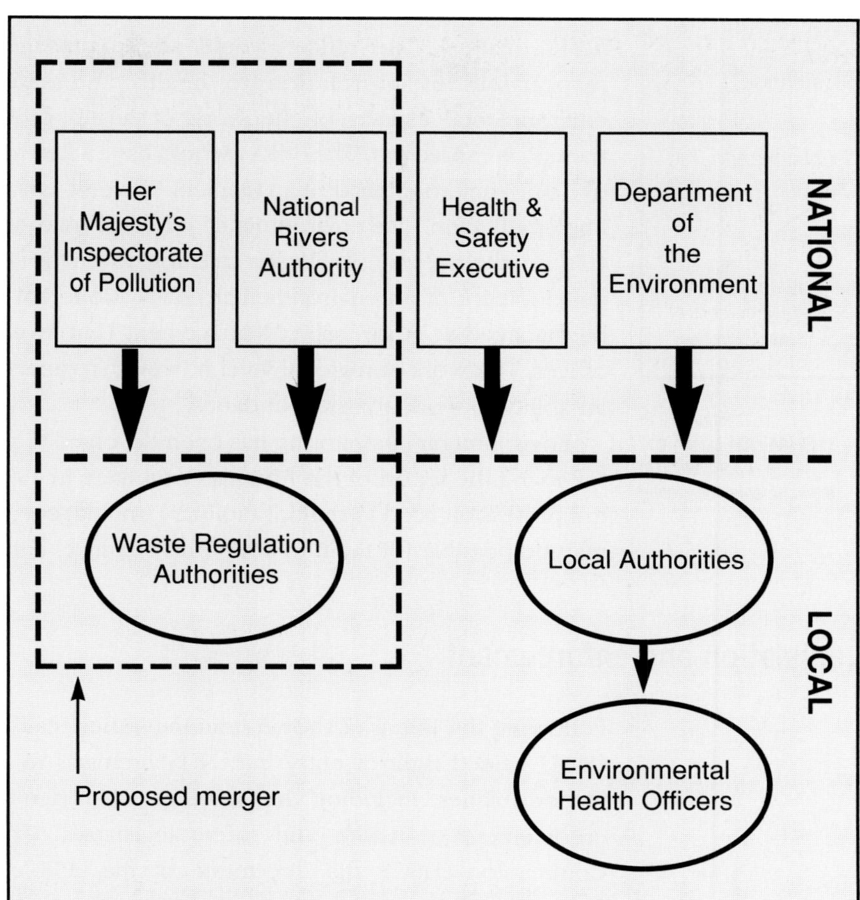

Figure 12.1: The present relationship between bodies regarding public and environmental health regulations and the proposed change

Environmental audit is currently undertaken on a voluntary basis. However, with responsibility and decision making devolved to local levels, it will become increasingly important to set clear national guidelines to be interpreted and acted upon locally. The NHS Executive should take the lead in this matter and thereby set the standards for individual health authorities and hospitals in the development of their own environmental management systems. The British Standard for Environmental Management (BS 7750) and the EC's Eco-Management and Audit Regulation (1993) both provide a generic framework for the monitoring of environmental performance. British Standard 7750 could be adopted as the NHS standard for environmental management systems; the targets to be achieved locally should be agreed by the Executive's regional offices, working with the designated environmental officer in each provider unit. The development of environmental management policies will need to reflect the national strategy for the environment, established by the proposed Environment Agency and current legislation, as advised by the Health Services Advisory Committee, and the Occupational Health Advisory Committee.

To provide coherent local action, every trust and directly managed unit should appoint or designate an environmental officer. The officer would act as a focus for the overlapping roles of many specialties such as occupational health, infection control, and communicable diseases, in environmental

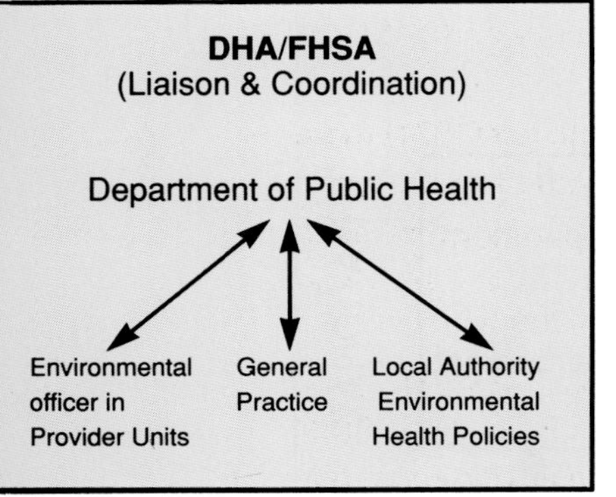

Figure 12.2: DHA/FHSA liaison and coordination in environmental monitoring

health matters. The officer would advise managers and staff of their responsibilities in relation to health and safety, co-ordinate the environmental aspects of the work of health professionals and ensure training is carried out. The officer would have a key role in the development of local environmental management systems and in monitoring their implementation. The environmental officer should be a source of advice to GPs on their responsibilities in relation to environmental health and on development of an environmental policy. Coherent local action may well be managed at Trust/District Management Unit level by an environmental officer. The work at regional level however, requires greater expertise and an ability to work across boundaries.

Environmental monitoring has been devolved to public health medicine following the report of the Abrams Committee in 1993[9] and as a branch of the profession used to multidisciplinary, multiagency collaborative work, it may be possible for them to adopt this strategic, liaison role. (Figure 12.2)

Legislation and enforcement

Following the lifting of Crown immunity, the Health and Safety Executive (HSE) gained right of entry into NHS premises to discharge its statutory responsibilities, including the provision of advice to employers and the enforcement of health and safety legislation. The Health and Safety Commission (HSC), the directorate of the HSE established the Health Services Advisory Committee and the Occupational Health Advisory Committee in line with their new responsibilities. The Health Services Advisory Committee, which consists of representatives from various parts of the health sector, including trade unions, advises the Health and Safety Commission on the implementation of regulations, guidance and EC directives within the health sector. The Health Services Advisory Committee also advises the HSE on its guidance to health authorities, aimed at helping them fulfil their responsibilities in occupational and environmental health and safety. The Health Services Advisory Committee advises the Health and Safety Commission on the health of people in all sectors of work. While continuing within its present remit, the Occupational Health Advisory Committee should lend its expertise to the NHS Executive to develop guidance specific to the health sector on occupational health services.

The agencies that are involved in assessing legislation and compliance are currently under-resourced and have too few staff to provide sufficient expertise in all areas, either to monitor effectively or to ensure offenders are prosecuted where necessary.[10] The main thrust of the work of the HSE is currently to control hazards in the workplace and its influence on protecting the general public is quite limited. It is therefore of great concern that the Government plans to reduce expenditure on the HSC by £5 million in 1994-1995 and £10 million in 1995-1996, with a cash freeze thereafter.[11] Further resources are required by the HSC is to fulfil its role in protecting both employees and the public from the hazards of work processes and if

the improvements seen since the introduction of the Health and Safety at Work etc Act (1974) are to be maintained and furthered.

Since promulgation of the Health and Safety at Work etc Act (1974) there has been a continuous flow of important legislation relating to health and safety at work and in the environment. While essential to ensuring the health and safety of the nation's workforce, these regulations are complex and numerous and require review.

The Health and Safety Commission has been requested to undertake a review of health and safety legislation as the Government is concerned that it may represent a burden on business. However, the real burden is that arising from accidents and disease, and on the environment, which legislation is designed to prevent. In fact there is a pressing need for a review of legislation, to ensure that there is comprehensive coverage of employees and the public alike. This is particularly true for the health care sector. The Health Services Advisory Committee should review legislation that affects the health care sector. The outcomes of the review would need to be widely disseminated to all those representing health care workers and to those with a role in health and safety aspects of the health care services, particularly if any changes in current legislation are proposed. A review would enable the development of appropriate occupational and environmental policies by the NHS Executive and by managers in the independent and private sector.

Information and research

Adequate information about the various hazards associated with health care and medical technology is needed. This report has revealed the inadequacy of information on the operational aspects of environmental and occupational health and the scarcity of epidemiological research. In addition, where the results of research are available these are frequently not disseminated nor applied. However, new medical technology and health care processes require rigorous assessment *before* their introduction to identify and control any potential risks in advance. These problems must be addressed before the health sector can effectively remedy the weaknesses of its environmental and occupational health policies. The HSE maintain a database of over 500,000 workplaces which inspectors use to plan their site visits, and 1,500 inspectors are grouped into seven separate inspectorates, covering: Factories, Agriculture, Nuclear, Offshore, Mines, Railways and Quarries. The HSE recognise that employers fail to report two-thirds of accidents and that under-reporting is a particular problem in relation to occupational ill health.[12]

The BMA's report on *The Morbidity and Mortality of the Medical Profession*[13] concluded that considerable research is required both to review existing sources of information and to undertake new prospective longitudinal studies of health care worker populations. Review of existing information could be carried out by a clearing house, set up to establish what we already know about the trends of death and illness within the profession. New research should be undertaken to fill in the gaps.

Occupational health physicians should keep detailed information by specialty on occupation-related illness to enable comparisons to be made of mortality and morbidity among medical practitioners and other groups. Data collection should include the taking of detailed occupational histories, confirmation of adverse effects resulting from chemical, radiation and biological exposures as well as workloads and other factors. However, general practitioners have an equal, if not greater, role in identifying occupationally related morbidity and mortality as they will attend to the health problems of a far greater section of the community than occupational health doctors.

The Health and Safety Executive, in order to improve the identification and treatment of occupationally acquired illness and injury, has circulated a guide to occupational health to all GPs.[14] General practitioners are encouraged to discuss confidentially, suspected occupational illness or injury, with the relevant occupational health department, to gain appropriate advice and to assist in the maintenance of occupational health records. General practitioners also have a vital role in identifying morbidity and mortality that could be related to environmental factors. The detailed recording of information and collation of results by general practitioners and occupational health doctors is necessary in order to identify preventable deaths and illness and enable proper assessment of the impact of medical technology and health care processes on patients, staff and the environment.

With the HSE, the NHS Research and Development Directorate should review the need for research into occupational and environmental problems in health care and consider this issue as a priority area for funding. The Occupational Health Advisory Committee and Health Services Advisory Committee along with individual occupational health departments could act as sources of advice about the need for research into existing, and newly emerging, occupational and environmental problems in the NHS.

A central database of research undertaken in this area should be established through the NHS Research and Development Directorate with the results widely disseminated throughout the health service. The central database will enable the NHS to issue guidance to local units based on currently available research evidence. Where research reveals a need for new or revised legislation, the HSC would advise the NHSE and Department of Health.

Infection control

Even though procedures for infection control are well established today, at least 1 in 20 of all hospital patients will pick up some form of infection whilst undergoing treatment. Hospital infection control committees perform a major role in the protection and education of staff, in surveillance of procedures, and reduction of nosocomial infections, and are therefore essential.

The Public Health Laboratory Service provides support for the diagnosis, prevention and control of infections and communicable diseases in England

and Wales. Its regional and area laboratories assist in the investigation of communicable disease problems in their locality, working closely with consultants in communicable disease control, and environmental health officers, local GPs and others involved in community health. The Communicable Disease Surveillance Centre is the national centre for surveillance of infectious and communicable disease. Working closely with area and regional public health laboratories it collects, analyses, and disseminates data on the occurrence and spread of communicable diseases it also provides assistance in the field with the investigation and management of major outbreaks.

Patients, staff, medical instruments, and health care buildings can all act as reservoirs for micro-organisms and as potential sources of infection. A variety of pathogens can cause serious infection. For staff, hepatitis B infection continues to be a major hazard and the risk of HIV or hepatitis C infection from needlestick injury or blood exposure, although small, is real. The risk of transmitting HIV from health care workers to patients appears to be minimal and it should be emphasised that doctors are at much greater risk from HIV-positive patients, than are patients from HIV-positive doctors. Mycobacteria which have developed multiple resistance to drugs present a risk to health care staff of contracting tuberculosis. Outbreaks due to multi drug resistant strains have been reported in hospitals in other countries[15-17] but no outbreaks are known to have occurred in the UK.[18] Several surveys of general practices in the UK have revealed uncertainty about procedures to control infection, with many practices lacking an infection control policy, leaving staff with inadequate information on which to make risk assessment decisions. Effective infection control policies are essential to prevent patient-to-patient transmission via contaminated surgical instruments. GPs have a legal obligation under the Health and Safety at Work etc Act (1974) to ensure that all their employees are appropriately trained and proficient in the procedures necessary for working safely, and they have a responsibility to protect voluntary workers. Furthermore, GPs are required by the Control of Substances Hazardous to Health (COSHH) Regulations (1988), to review every procedure carried out by their employees which involves contact with a substance, hazardous to health, including pathogenic micro-organisms. However, doctors and practice nurses may not have received formal training in the safe use and disposal of sharps and should consider adopting guidelines such as the BMA's *Code of Practice for the Safe Use and Disposal of Sharps*[19] and *Code of Practice for Sterilisation of Instruments and Control of Cross-Infection*[20] as recommended by the Department of Health[21] and the Health and Safety Executive.[22]

The Department of Health has issued guidelines which advise all health care workers who perform 'exposure prone procedures', including independent contractors such as GPs and dentists, to be immunised against hepatitis B. However, these guidelines should be strengthened to require health service employers to provide immunisation for all staff and students who are in frequent contact with blood and sharps.[23] Occupational health personnel have a central role in implementing staff immunisation

programmes and monitoring occupational health. With an effective immunisation programme, the risk to staff from HBV will be greatly reduced. It will be important that the system of immunisation is introduced smoothly, with correct policies for dealing with any problems that arise, such as the situation in which individuals fail to sero-convert and therefore remain at risk from hepatitis B infection. However, a more recently recognised infection risk is that caused by the hepatitis C virus for which no vaccine is available, so protection from this agent and also HIV, will still depend on staff strictly following safe working practices.

Clinical waste

The problems associated with the disposal of waste were examined in the BMA's 1991 report *Hazardous Waste and Human Health.*[24] Currently the total waste arising from premises owned and operated by health authorities or NHS trusts in the UK, classified as clinical waste, exceeds 155,000 tonnes per annum. In addition, independent hospitals, GPs, dentists, nursing/residential homes and blood transfusion centres create a further 70,000 tonnes annually.

Clinical waste is composed of many different constituents which vary widely in the hazards they present. (see box on page 129)

Segregation and management systems can recover glass, plastic, metal and paper containers from health care products, as well as packaging used for transportation or protection. Manufacturers should be encouraged by NHS purchasers to design recyclable products, especially packaging.

The most hazardous components of the clinical waste stream are sharps — used needles, blades and other similar items. Unless they are disposed of correctly, in appropriate British Standard quality containers, there is a real risk of injury and possible transmission of infection, particularly with blood borne pathogens such as HIV and viral hepatitis. The Department of Environment Waste Management Paper No. 25 (currently under revision)[25] recommends that sharps containers should have a British Standard kite mark and, where practical, conform to BS 7320 (1990) or its equivalent.

Clinical waste management

Effective waste management should be carried out in three main stages:

- The risk assessment of the components of the waste stream.
- The segregation of waste according to its relative risks enabling appropriate disposal or recovery for recycling.
- The minimisation of waste, through the use of disposable items only where essential and by encouraging the use of recyclable products.

The effective training of a wide spectrum of health care staff in the management of waste can only be organised and managed if there is a central training function within each hospital, health authority or trust. Priority must be given to the training of health care workers particularly in the safe handling of sharps. In all hospitals infection control committees should ensure that a professional member of staff is appointed as a training officer and allocated to this task. Accepted codes of practice, such as the BMA's,[26,27] should be made freely available to all those handling sharps and clinical waste.

Incineration is currently the main method of disposal of clinical waste. With the loss of Crown immunity and the introduction of the Environmental Protection Act (1990), stringent standards have been set for all incinerator plants in the NHS. These must be met within a two-stage deadline by 1995. Unless the Government provides all hospitals with extra funding to ensure that their incineration capacity reaches the required standards by this deadline, clinical waste will have to be transported long distances by private waste disposal contractors which may be unsuitable and will certainly be very costly. The safe destruction of all sharps and other high risk clinical waste items on-site, within the hospital, is preferable.

The NHS Executive should ensure that NHS managers are kept informed of the Health and Safety Executive's guidance, of their liability in law, revised guidance from the Department of the Environment, together with the advice of professional bodies and ensure that only the safest and most appropriate system for clinical waste disposal is followed.

Health care building design

With the removal of Crown immunity the NHS needs to be certain of its compliance with statutory health and safety requirements which affect NHS properties. The NHS Estates Agency provides safety notices on health and safety matters and acts as a focal point for liaison with the Health and Safety Executive, where there are defects and failures in plant equipment and buildings. Such guidance is essential reading for architects, managers, planning teams, NHS trust chief executives and FHSAs, who should ensure that all plans for new or refurbished health care buildings take account of guidance given by the NHS Estates Agency.

All NHS properties should be subject to a building and design audit to ensure compliance with both legislation and the NHS Estates Agency guidelines. Existing NHS buildings must keep pace with developing medical technology and information obtained from audit and outcome measurement should be used to ensure that existing buildings are maintained to the highest standards; extra funding to the NHS may be required to ensure the maximum compliance with such audits.

The quality factor

The Department of Health is committed to ensuring that the health service is well managed and that resources are used efficiently. The overall objectives of the NHS are, "promoting health, preventing disease and providing high quality services and patient care". Following the 1991 programme of reforms in the NHS there is now a further programme of change, which is summarised in the recently published document *Managing the New NHS.*[28] This document reports the results of a review body which was set up in May 1993 to examine the structure, functions and manpower required to complete the series of NHS reforms. Government has decided that the effectiveness of the NHS in delivering services to patients would be improved by streamlining the central management structure and consolidating joint working, between District Health Authorities and Family Health Services Authorities. This would involve reorganising the NHS Executive through abolition of the fourteen statutory Regional Health Authorities, and the seven NHS outposts, and replacement with eight regional offices. The District Health Authorities and Family Health Services Authorities will merge to create stronger local purchasers, furthering the drive towards decentralisation.

Managing the New NHS provides a focus for the management of human resources which will flow from the further reforms, but fails to set quality standards for the health and safety of NHS employees. It is not enough to say simply that, "staff [should] work as efficiently as possible in the interest of patient safety and good quality care".[29] The philosophy of this further reorganisation must ensure that the safety of staff is given a high priority, through the establishment of an occupational health service for all NHS employees, and meaningful policing of legislation.

Successive Annual Representative Meetings of the BMA have passed resolutions on occupational health in the NHS, requesting assurances from the NHS Executive that the new statutory obligations coming into force early in 1993 regarding health and safety would be acted upon — but little progress has been achieved. The establishment of an occupational health service is essential in addressing the risks of health care processes outlined in this report, to the public, patients, environment and health care workers. The Association, although supporting the 1992 publication *Health at Work in the NHS*, was concerned at the suggested timetable for review of health and safety practice.

The Government should now ensure that the *Health at Work in the NHS* initiative is acted upon immediately, to introduce a systematic healthy work-place programme throughout the NHS. Resources and support should be provided for implementing policies for smoking cessation, healthy eating, stress management, sensible drinking and in promoting exercise. AIDS and infection control awareness days should be organised to ensure that staff are aware of the social and occupational risks of HIV and other infections. Such events would provide the opportunity to reinforce staff awareness

about good clinical waste management and the need to consider economy and recycling wherever possible.

As a professional body the BMA does much in the way of advising and supporting doctors and their colleagues in matters related to their health and safety and the environment. It is clear however, that the profession needs a nationally organised initiative, implemented at local level to raise standards. It is in the interests of patients that the health needs of health care workers are given high priority, and in the interests of the public that health care managers address the environmental effects of health care processes. It is proposed that 1995 should be the National Health Service Year of Safety, Health and Hygiene at work, and this should be a major objective within the Government's proposals for the 'new' NHS.

Recommendations

1. **National policies on the environment**
   The National Environment Agency should be established without further delay. The powers and remit of the proposed Agency should be considered carefully, so that it will be able to address effectively environmental issues in relation to the health care services.

   The NHS Executive should take full responsibility for managing the effects of the NHS workplace on the wider environment, by establishing a comprehensive environmental policy for the NHS.

2. **Local policies on the environment**
   Every hospital or unit should appoint an environmental officer or manager with responsibility for co-ordinating environmental health and to assist in the development of local environmental policies. The environmental officer should liaise with the District Health Authority/Family Health Service Authority and the Department of Public Health Medicine, who may take on a strategic, liaison role in the organisation of NHS environmental policies.

   The establishment of coherent environmental policies should be a pre-requisite for approval of trust status and should be required in all private hospitals in the UK.

3. **Health at work in the NHS**
   The Department of Health through the National Health Service Executive should set quality standards for health and safety and environmental health for NHS employees, to be achieved by the end of 1995.

   The NHS Executive must establish a consultant-led occupational health service as a matter of urgency, to meet the needs of all those working in the health care sector, including general medical and dental practices. The provision of an occupational health service should be a pre-requisite for approval of trust status and should be required in all private hospitals.

All health care workers should be trained in infection control and the safe use and disposal of sharps.

All health care workers who are in frequent contact with body fluids and sharps, including independent contractors — such as GP's and dentists working outside the hospital setting, and all medical, dental, nursing and midwifery students should be immunised against hepatitis B.

General practitioners should ensure that their practice has an infection control policy, with adequate reporting and follow-up procedures, in the event of sharps injury or blood exposure.

Confidential, voluntary HIV testing should be available for health care workers through a consultant-led occupational health service.

4. Education

All NHS staff should be trained to identify, report and prevent hazards in the health service to a level appropriate to their activities and responsibilities.

Undergraduate and postgraduate medical education should include environmental awareness and training in health and safety.

Occupational physicians and nurses should be provided with specialist training in environmental health. Further training and education in environmental health should be available to public health doctors.

5. Information

A national database on environmental and occupational health should be established through the NHS Research and Development Directorate and made available to health service managers and staff, particularly environmental officers and occupational health professionals.

The NHS Research and Development Directorate should co-ordinate new research into the various hazards associated with health care and medical technology with government departments, the Research Councils and Universities.

6. Management of clinical waste

The risks posed by the various components of the clinical waste stream should be regularly assessed. This can then form the basis of an appropriate, safe and cost effective national strategy of waste management within the NHS, taking account of developing technology.

The policy for handling the increasing volume of waste generated through general practice and home visits should be reviewed in conjunction with the local FHSA.

Resources should be earmarked to ensure a national network of modern incinerators accessible by all health care units producing clinical waste. This should be backed by appropriate national regulations that include regular monitoring of waste disposal.

7. **Legislation and enforcement**

Further resources are needed by the Health and Safety Commission for it to fulfil its role in protecting both workers and the public from hazards in the work place.

The Health and Safety Commission should undertake a review of the health and safety legislation covering the health care sector and publish their findings.

All NHS properties should be subject to a building and design audit to ensure compliance with legislation and NHS Estates Agency guidelines and government targets for energy savings.

APPENDIX I
Sources of information

Professional Organisations

British Occupational Hygiene Society: Suite 2, Georgian House, Great Northern Road, Derby DE1 1LT.

Chartered Institution of Building Services: (incorporating what were formerly the Institution of Heating and Ventilation Engineers and the Illuminating Engineering Society), Delta House, 222 Balham High Road, London SW12 9BS.

English National Board for Nursing, Midwifery and Health Visiting: Victory House, 170 Tottenham Court Road, London W1P 0HA.

Ergonomics Society: Dept Human Sciences, University of Technology, Loughborough LE11 3TU.

Faculty of Occupational Medicine: Royal College of Physicians, 6 St Andrew's Place, London NW1 4LE.

Faculty of Public Medicine: 4 St Andrews Place, London NW1 4LB.

Institute of Occupational Hygienists: Suite 2, Georgian House, Great Northern Road, Derby DE1 1LT.

Institute of Occupational Safety and Health: 222 Uppingham Road, Leicester LE5 0QG.

APPENDIX II
Training and education

There are a number of courses and examinations available in the UK which offer training and professional qualifications in occupational and environmental health and related topics. Listed below are some examples.

Faculty of Occupational Medicine

The Faculty has an important role in promoting training in occupational medicine. In each NHS region, Regional Specialty Advisers and Deputies have been appointed jointly by the Faculty and the Joint Committee on Higher Medical Training. Advisers have an important role in postgraduate training at regional and district level.

The Faculty admits Associates and Members, and Fellows of the Faculty may be elected by the Board. The Diploma of Associateship (AFOM) is a qualification available to those medical practitioners who have sufficient broad clinical experience and full or part-time experience in Occupational Medicine satisfying the Regulations, and who pass the examination for the Associateship of the Faculty of Occupational Medicine. The Diploma of Membership (MFOM) is intended for registered medical practitioners who wish to become specialists in occupational medicine. In 1994, a diploma in occupational medicine will be introduced which will be available to medical practitioners, with a limited or part-time interest in the practice of occupational medicine. They will follow a faculty approved training course and take an examination arranged by the Faculty of Occupational Medicine.

Faculty of Public Health Medicine

Training in public health medicine involves at least seven years at general professional, basic specialist levels; to gain membership of the Faculty of Public Health Medicine, which is a Faculty of the Royal College of

Physicians. Doctors enter at registrar level and progress to senior registrar. They may do an MSc during the training period or via consortium arrangements which leads to Part 1 of the membership examination. Part 2 is awarded following presentation of a satisfactory dissertation and *viva voce* examination. Some of the subjects covered during training include epidemiology, communicable disease, environmental health and health service planning and evaluation.

Institute of Occupational Hygienists

The constitution of the Institute is aimed at maintaining a high standard of professional practice in occupational hygiene. Membership is open to practitioners who meet defined levels of experience and competence. The Institute is concerned with the promotion of study of, teaching and training in occupational hygiene. It supervises examinations and awards diplomas or certificates in occupational hygiene or allied subjects.

The British Examining Board of Occupational Hygiene (BEBOH) appraises the competence at various levels of ability of practising occupational hygienists. It governs Preliminary Certificate examinations including written and oral elements. It also awards Certificates and Diplomas to persons who satisfy the requirements. Professional accreditation is awarded by the Institute of Occupational Hygienists who consider practical experience and academic record based on either the BEBOH Preliminary Certificate, Certificate or Diploma, or acceptable equivalents together with the relevant BEBOH or IOH oral examination.

English National Board for Nursing, Midwifery and Health Visiting (ENB)

Gives formal approval of course and colleges leading to an occupational health and nursing qualifications. In addition to their nursing qualifications, nurses may take additional qualifications in occupational health. The qualification in occupational health nursing is the occupational health nursing certificate (OHNC). This is awarded by the English National Board for Nursing, Midwifery and Health Visiting after a period of training and the successful completion of an examination.

The Royal College of Nursing

The Royal College of Nursing awards a BSc in Health Studies (Occupational Health) which includes a set number of modules in occupational health. Also provides courses validated by the E.N.B.

The Robens Institute, University of Surrey

Provides postgraduate training in the following areas:-

Advanced Diploma/MSc course in Occupational Health and Safety

These courses are validated by ENB, BEBOH and IOSH, open to practitioners in the field of health and safety whatever their discipline.

The course is modular and requires attendance at the University plus home-based study.

Diploma in Occupational Medicine

Validated by the Faculty of Occupational Medicine of the Royal College of Physicians. This is a part-time day-release course open to medical practitioners working part-time in the practice of occupational medicine. It is not part of the formal training route to Membership and Specialist Accreditation.

MSc/Postgraduate Diploma in Applied Toxicology

The course is offered in the form of six modules per year and there is an option of completing the course by course work alone or by course work plus project. Each module is run on the University of Surrey campus as an intensive week of lectures, tutorials, case studies and demonstrations. Participants are also required to undertake prescribed reading at home and to submit a home assignment essay for each module. The successful completion of 12 modules or equivalent is required for the award of the MSc.

Modular MSc/Advanced Diploma/ Advanced Certificate in Environmental Management and Health

Offered jointly by the Robens Institute and Farnborough College of Technology. The programme is based on a series of intensive one week courses, supported by comprehensive distance learning material. Successful completion of four modules leads to an Advanced Certificate; successful completion of eight modules to an Advanced Diploma. A Masters degree can be achieved through one of two routes: (i) successful completion of twelve modules or (ii) successful completion of eight modules plus a dissertation and viva voce examination. All modules are individually assessed.

Glossary

absorbed dose of radiation: quantity of energy imparted by ionising radiation to a unit mass of matter such as tissue. Unit gray, symbol Gy. 1Gy=1joule per kilogram.

acute exposure: short term exposure to a substance, for instance, through an accident.

additive effects: an effect of two substances in combination which are equal to the sum of their individual effects.

aerosol: a dispersion of solid or liquid particles in a gas.

aetiology: the science of causation - particularly of a disease.

allergy: Acquired state of immunological hyper-sensitivity in humans and animals to allergens (substances foreign to the body) induced by exposure through injection, inhalation, ingestion or skin contact

Ames test: a test in which specific bacteria are used to assess whether a chemical will cause mutation of the genetic information (DNA) in the bacteria, helping predict whether the chemical may cause cancer in humans or animals.

amniocentesis: the withdrawal of amniotic fluid through the abdominal or vaginal wall by means of a syringe and needle to diagnose certain biochemical or chromosomal disorders of the foetus.

angioplasty: surgery within a blood vessel, usually by means of a balloon-tipped catheter.

antigen: a foreign substance such as a viral protein that causes the formation of antibodies

antimicrobial: a substance which destroys bacteria or inhibits their growth.

antisepsis: destruction of inhibition of the growth of bacteria (sufficient to prevent putrefication of disease).

asepsis: freedom from pathogenic micro-organisms.

autoclave: apparatus for sterilising materials by exposing them to steam in a closed vessel at a high temperature and pressure for a period of time.

barium enema/barium meal: a preparation, consisting mainly of barium sulphate (which is opaque to x-rays), administered as an enema or a meal to reveal abnormality in the stomach or intestines, and to show gut motility.

beta particle: an electron emitted by the nucleus of a radionuclide and which usually carries a negative charge. The electric charge may be positive, in which case the beta particle is called a positron.

bovine spongiform encephalopathy (BSE): a fatal, slow developing disease of cattle affecting the nervous system.

cannula: a hollow tube for insertion into the body by which fluids are introduced or removed.

carcinogenicity: the ability of a substance to cause cancer.

carcinogen: a cancer causing substance.

catheter: a rigid or flexible tube introduced into body cavities or organs, either for investigational purposed or for some form of treatment.

chlorofluorocarbons (CFCs): chlorine-based compounds used in the manufacture of aerosol propellants, refrigerants, and foam packaging. CFCs contribute to the 'greenhouse' effect and are also a factor in the depletion of the ozone layer.

chromosome: rod-shaped bodies which contain the genes, or hereditary elements. Humans possess 23 pairs and are found in the nucleus of every body cell.

chronic exposure: exposure over a prolonged period of time often of a low level, sometimes for the duration of a lifetime.

chronotropic: Affecting the speed of muscle contraction, (heart rate).

congenital malformations: abnormality of any portion or organ of the body that develops during pregnancy and which is present at birth.

cosmic rays: high energy ionising radiation from outer space.

cytostatic: a substance which suppresses cell growth at multiplication.

cytotoxic: harmful to cells and cell division.

diathermy: production of heat by a high frequency electric current.

dielectric: a non-conducting medium capable of transmitting an electrostatic charge by induction.

DNA - deoxyribonucleic acid: The compound, found in chromosomes that controls the structure and function of cells and is the material of inheritance.

dysaesthesia: abnormality in feeling or sense of touch.

electromagnetic fields: a field, of force equivalent to an electric field and a magnetic field at right angles to each other and to the direction of propagation.

epidemiology: The study of the distribution and determinants of disease in populations.

erythropoietin: a hormone produced by the kidney that stimulates the production of red blood cells in the bone marrow.

eugenics: the study of methods of improving the quality of the human race especially through selective breeding.

furans: name given to a number of chemicals (polychlorinated dibenzofurans) that may be produced during low temperature incineration and may be harmful to health.

gas-scavenging: removing excess anaesthetic gases from the operating theatre.

gene therapy: the replacement or repair of defective genes in living cells.

gram-negative, gram-positive: classificatory terms for two types of bacteria according to the ability of bacteria to retain the violet of Gram's stains. Those that do so are designated gram- positive, those that do not, gram-negative.

gray: the derived System International unit of absorbed ionising radiation dose equivalent to an absorption per unit mass of one joule per kilogram of irradiated material. Symbol: Gy.

greenhouse effect: the warming of the lower atmosphere outgoing radiation caused by reflection back from the earth's surface trapped by greenhouse gases such as CFCs, carbon dioxide, methane, nitrous oxide, and tropospheric ozone.

haemodialysis: dialysis of blood, as in kidney machines, to remove toxic chemicals.

haemoglobinopathy: a disease of the blood associated with the presence of an abnormal haemoglobin in the red blood cells.

half life: the time taken for the activity of a radionuclide to be reduced by 50% through decay.

hepatoxicity: ability to cause destruction of the liver cells.

hypersensitivity: abnormally heightened sensitivity to a foreign agent, small doses of which produce a violent reaction in a patient.

immunocompromised: have the immune response attenuated.

immunosuppressant drugs: drugs which induce suppression of the body's defence mechanism against infection and foreign substances, used in organ transplantation to prevent the body rejecting the transplanted organ.

intubation: the introduction of a tube, usually into the trachea to allow ventilation of the lungs. Used for the administration of an anaesthetic.

isotope: a nuclide of a particular chemical element with the same number of protons but different number of neutrons.

maceration: breaking down of solid waste.

mutagenicity: the property of a physical, chemical or biological agent to induce mutation in living cells, leading to inherited differences (mutation).

nebuliser: device for converting a liquid into a mist or fine spray.

neoplasm: a tumour or cancer - new growth.

nephrotoxicity: the ability of a substance to cause destruction of/or toxic action on the cells of the kidney.

neurophysiological: relating to the physiology of the nervous system.

neuropsychiatric: relating to nervous and mental disorders.

nosocomial infection: an infection acquired while in hospital.

ozone layer: concentration of the gas ozone in the stratosphere, it affords protection for the earth against harmful ultraviolet radiation from the sun.

parenteral nutrition: nutrition introduced into the body by routes other than the mouth eg intravenously or subcutaneously.

photo-chemical smog: a form of pollution found in heavily motorised cities produced by chemical reactions particularly between nitrogen oxides and hydrocarbons, under the influence of sunlight.

plasmid: a small circular piece of DNA found in some bacteria which replicates independently of the main bacterial DNA.

prion: small infectious particles of protein found in brain tissue of humans and other species suffering from spongiform encephalopathy such as scrapie in sheep or Creutzfeldt-Jakob disease.

prophylactic: an agent used to prevent disease.

radioisotope: an unstable isotope which decays to a stable state by emitting characteristic radiation. Usually the substance is an element which has been made radioactive by artificial means.

radionuclide: an unstable nuclide that emits ionising radiation.

radiotherapy: treatment of disease by radium, x-rays or radioactive isotopes.

sensitisation: a condition in which the response to a second and subsequent stimuli is greater than to the original stimulus; the immune process by which individuals become hypersensitive to such substances as pollen, animal dander (see hypersensitivity).

sharps: anything that can puncture the skin including hypodermic and suture needles and blades, sharp bones and broken glass.

sievert: the derived Systme International unit of dose, equivalent to 1 joule per kilogram. Symbol: Sv.

somatic cells: all body cells except sexual reproductive cells.

stoma bag: a bag attached to the abdominal wall to collect excreta from a stoma following a colostomy, ileostomy or urostomy.

synergistic: phenomenon in which the effect produced by two (or more) substances together, is greater than the sum of the effects produced by the substances separately.

systemic: pertaining to the body as a whole rather than its individual parts.

teratogenicity: the ability of a substance or condition to cause deviations from normal growth and development between conception and birth, resulting in abnormal individuals.

tomography: special imaging technique used in radiology to record internal body images at a predetermined plane.

transudate: any fluid which passes through a membrane.

venepuncture: the insertion of a needle into a vein, usually to obtain a blood specimen.

in vitro fertilisation: fertilisation carried out outside the body under laboratory conditions.

References

Introduction

1. NHS Estates. A strategic guide to environment policy for general managers and chief executives. London: NHS Estates, 1992.
2. Department of Environment. Sustainable development: the UK strategy. (Cmnd 2426). London: HMSO, 1994
3. British Medical Association. A code of practice for the safe use and disposal of sharps. London: BMA, 1990.
4. British Medical Association. A code of practice for sterilisation of instruments and control of cross infection. London: BMA, 1989.
5. British Medical Association. Hazardous waste and human health. Oxford: OUP, 1991.
6. British Medical Association. The BMA guide to pesticides, chemicals and health. (2nd ed.) London: Edward Arnold, 1992.
7. British Medical Association. Cycling: towards health and safety. Oxford: OUP, 1992

CHAPTER 1

1. Szreter S. The importance of social intervention in Britain's mortality decline c. 1850-1914: a re-interpretation of the role of public health. Social History of Medicine 1988;1:1-37.
2. Rhodes P. An outline history of medicine. London: Butterworths, 1985.
3. Editorial. The Lancet 1871;2:266.

4. Davy H. Researches, chemical and philosophical, chiefly concerning nitrous oxide, or dephlogisticated nitrous air and its respiration. London: J Johnson, 1800.

5. Kirschner M. Zur hygiene des operationssales. Zentralbl Chir 1925;52:2162-2165.

6. Perthes G. Shutz der am operationstischbeschaftigten vor schadigungdurch die narkosegase. Zentralbl Chir 1925;52:852-854.

7. Vaisman AI. Working conditions in surgery and their effect on the health of anaesthesiologists. Eksp Khir Anestheziol 1967;3:44- 49.

8. Minutes of the Anaesthetics in Midwifery Committee, 1929-1930, BMA Archive.

9. Bleich AR. The story of x-rays from Röntgen to isotopes. New York: Dover Publications Inc, 1960.

10. ibid.

11. Moodie I. The Society of Radiographers, 50 years of history. London: Society of Radiographers, 1969.

12. Kipling M. A brief history of HM Medical Inspectorate. London: HSE, 1979.

13. Dixon WM, Price SMG. Aspects of occupational health. London: Faber, 1984.

14. Control of substances hazardous to health regulations. SI 1657. London: HMSO, 1988.

15. Myers JA. Tuberculosis, a half century of study and conquest. Lewis S E, Green WH. 1970: 166-99, quoted in Goldman KP. Tuberculosis in Hospital Doctors. Tubercle 1988;69:237-240.

16. Nosocomial infection surveillance. MMWR CDC surveillance summary 35. (No.1 s17ss). 1986.

CHAPTER 2

1. Royal commission on environmental pollution. Twelth report. Best practicable environmental option. London: HMSO, 1988.

2. British Medical Association. Living with risk. (2nd ed.) London: Penguin, 1990.

3. Richardson ML ed. Risk assessment of chemicals in the environment. London: Royal Society of Chemistry, 1988.

4. Amdur MO. Air pollutants. In: Klaassen CD, Amdur MO, Doull J, ed. Casarett and Doull's Toxicology. (3rd ed.) New York: MacMillan, 1986:801-824

5. WHO. Air quality guidelines for Europe, WHO Regional Publications, European series. No 23. Copenhagen: WHO Regional Office for Europe, 1987.

6. ibid.

7. Department of Health. Ozone. Advisory group on the medical aspects of air pollution episodes. London: HMSO, 1991.

8. Amdur MO. Air pollutants. In: Klaassen CD, Amdur MO, Doull J, ed. Casarett and Doull's Toxicology. (3rd ed.) New York: MacMillan, 1986:801-824.

9. Harrison RM ed. Pollution, causes, effects and control. (2nd ed.) London: Royal Society of Chemistry, 1990.

10. ibid.

11. WHO. Indoor air quality: organic pollutants. Report of a WHO meeting. EURO Reports and Studies 111. Copenhagen: WHO, Regional Office for Europe, 1989.

12. WHO. Air quality guidelines for Europe, WHO Regional Publications, European series. No 23. Copenhagen: WHO Regional Office for Europe, 1987.

13. Harrison RM ed. Pollution, causes, effects and control. (2nd ed.) London: Royal Society of Chemistry, 1990.

14. Dayan AD. Carcinogenicity and drinking water. Phamacol Toxicol 1993 72, Suppl 1:S108-115.

15. ECETOC. Concentrations of industrial chemicals measured in the environment. Technical Report No 29. Brussels: ECETOC, 1988.

16. Ward S, May G, Heath A et al. Carbaryl metabolism is inhibited by cimetidine in the isolated perfused rat liver and man. J. Toxicol Clin Toxicol 1968;26:551-555.

17. Rider J A, Moeller H C, Swader J, Devereaux R G. A study of the anticholinesterase properties of EPN and malathion in human volunteers. Clin Res 1959;7:81-2.

18. British Medical Association. The BMA guide to pesticides, chemicals and health. (2nd ed.) London: Edward Arnold, 1992.

19. Brain JD, Beck BD, Warren AJ, Shaikh RA. Variations in susceptibility to inhaled pollutants. Baltimore: Johns Hopkins UP, 1988.

20. WHO. Air quality guidelines for Europe, WHO Regional Publications, European series. No 23. Copenhagen: WHO Regional Office for Europe, 1987.

21. Department of Health. Ozone. Advisory group on the medical aspects of air pollution episodes. London: HMSO, 1991.

22. Burr ML. Epidemiology of asthma. In: Burr ML, ed. Epidemiology of Clinical Allergy. Basle: Monogr Allergy, 1993;31:80-102.

23. Department of Health. Ozone. Advisory group on the medical aspects of air pollution episodes. London: HMSO, 1991.

24. WHO. Air quality guidelines for Europe, WHO Regional Publications, European series. No 23. Copenhagen: WHO Regional Office for Europe, 1987.

25. Royal Commission on Environmental Pollution. 1988. Best practicable environmental option. 12th Report. (Cmnd 310). London: HMSO, 1988.

26. Cairncross F. Costing the earth. London: Economist Books, 1991.

27. OECD. Environmental policy. How to apply economic instruments. Paris: OECD, 1991.

28. WHO. Air quality guidelines for Europe, WHO Regional Publications, European series. No 23. Copenhagen: WHO Regional Office for Europe, 1987.

29. Macrory R. The legal control of pollution. In: Harrison RM, op. cit. 1990:277-297.

30. UK Government. This common inheritance. Britain's environmental strategy. (Cmnd 1200). London: HMSO, 1990.

CHAPTER 3

1. HSE. Occupational exposure limits, EH40-1994. London: HMSO, 1994.

2. Information based on a personal communication from M Campbell, Occupational Hygienist, Institute of Occupational Health, University of Birmingham

3. Adams RM ed. Occupational skin disease. (2nd ed.). Philadelphia: WB Saunders Company, 1990.

4. Martin PA, Cross HJ, Harrington JM. Formaldehyde: a report. Birmingham: IOH, 1986.

5. Hathaway GJ, Proctor NH, Hughes JP, Fischman ML. Proctor and Hughes' chemical hazards of the workplace. (3rd ed.) New York: Van Nostrand Reinhold, 1991.

6. Olsen JH, Dossing M. Formaldehyde induced symptoms in day care centers. Am Ind Hyg Assoc J 1982;43:366- 370.

7. Kilburn KH, Seidman BC, Warshaw R. Neurobehavioural and respiratory symptoms of formaldehyde and xylene exposure in histology technicians. Arch Env Health 1985;40:229-233.

8. Olsen JH, Dossing M. Formaldehyde induced symptoms in day care centers. Am Ind Hyg Assoc J 1982;43:366-370.

9. Kilburn KH, Seidman BC, Warshaw R. Neurobehavioural and respiratory symptoms of formaldehyde and xylene exposure in histology technicians. Arch Env Health 1985;40:229-233.

10. Norback D, Ingegerd M, Widstrom J. Indoor air quality and personal factors related to the sick building syndrome. Scand J Work Environ Health 1990;16:121-8.

11. Skov P, Valbjorn O, Pedersen BV. Influence of indoor climate on the sick building syndrome in an office environment. Scand J Work Environ Health 1990;16:363-71.

12. Kilburn KH, Seidman BC, Warshaw R. Neurobehavioural and respiratory symptoms of formaldehyde and xylene exposure in histology technicians. Arch Env Health 1985;40:229-233.

13. Hendrick DJ, Lane DJ. Formalin asthma in hospital staff. Br Med J 1975;i:607-8.

14. Hendrick DJ, Lane DJ. Occupational formalin asthma. Br J Ind Med 1977;34:11-18.

15. Burge PS, Harries MG, Lam WK, O'Brien IM, Patchett PA. Occupational asthma due to formaldehyde. Thorax 1985;40:255-260.

16. Harving H, Korsgaard J, Dahl R, Pedersen OF, Molhave L. Low concentrations of formaldehyde in bronchial asthma. Br Med J 1986;293:310.

17. Witek TJ, Schachter EN, Tosun T, Beck GJ, Leaderer BP. An evaluation of respiratory effects following exposure to 2.0ppm formaldehyde in asthmatics: lung function, symptoms, and airway reactivity. Arch Environ Health 1987;42:230-237.

18. Hathaway GJ, Proctor NH, Hughes JP, Fischman ML. Proctor and Hughes' chemical hazards of the workplace. (3rd ed.) New York: Van Nostrand Reinhold, 1991.

19. Gestal JJ. Occupational hazards in hospitals: accidents, radiation, exposure to noxious chemicals, drug addiction and psychic problems, and assault. Br J Ind Med 1987;44:510-520.

20. ibid.

21. Swenberg JA, Kerns WD, Mitchell RJ, Gralla EJ, Pavkov KL. Inductions of squamous cell carcinoma of the rat nasal cavity by inhalation exposure to formaldehyde vapour. Cancer Res 1980;40:3398-3402.

22. Kers W et al. Carcinogenicity of formaldehyde in rats and mice after long-term inhalation exposure. Cancer Res 1983;43:4382- 4392.

23. Batelle Columbus Laboratories. Final report on a chronic inhalation toxicology study in rats and mice exposed to formaldehyde. CIIT 1981:31.

24. Thomson EJ, Shackleton S, Harrington JM. Chromosome aberrations and sister-chromatid exchange frequencies in pathology staff occupationally exposed to formaldehyde. Mutation Res 1984;141:89-93.

25. Harrington JM, Shannon HS. Mortality study of pathologists and medical laboratory technicians. Br Med J 1975;ii:329-332.

26. Harrington JM, Oakes D. Mortality study of British pathologists 1974-80. Br J Ind Med 1984;41:188-191.

27. Hall A, Harrington JM, Aw TC. Mortality study of British pathologists. Am J Ind Med 1991;20:83-89.

28. IARC monographs suppl 7, 1987:211-216.

29. International Agency for Research on Cancer. Overall evaluations of carcinogenicity: an update of IARC monographs volumes 1-42. IARC monographs on the evaluation of carcinogenic risk to humans. Supplement 7, WHO: Léon, France, 1987.

30. Kilburn KH, Seidman BC, Warshaw R. Neurobehavioural and respiratory symptoms of formaldehyde and xylene exposure in histology technicians. Arch Env Health 1985;40:229-233.

31. Skisak CM. Formaldehyde vapour exposures in anatomy laboratories. Am Ind Hyg Assoc J 1983;44:948-950.

32. Coldiron VR, Ward JB, Trieff NM, Janssen HE, Smith JH. Occupational exposure to formaldehyde in a medical centre autopsy service. J Occup Med 1983;25:544-548.

33. Daniels WJ. Health hazard evaluation report, No HETA 89- 007-1983, St Thomas More Hospital, Canyon City, Colorado. Cincinnati, Ohio: NIOSH, 1989

34. Smith KA, Williams PL, Middendorf PJ, Zakraysek N. Kidney dialysis: ambient formaldehyde levels. Am Ind Hyg Assoc 1984;45:48-50.

35. Anonymous. Formaldehyde exposure in dialysis units. Dialysis and transplantation 1983;12:43- 44.

36. Elliott L. Walk through survey of the dialysis unit in a hospital in Cincinnati, Ohio, to evaluate exposure to formaldehyde. Cincinnati, Ohio: NIOSH,1982.

37. Information based on a personal communication from M Campbell, Occupational Hygienist, Institute of Occupational Health, University of Birmingham

38. Jachuk SJ, Bound CL, Steel J, Blain PG. Occupational hazard in hospital staff exposed to 2 per cent glutaraldehyde in an endoscopy unit. J Soc Occup Med 1989;39:69-71.

39. Norback D. Skin and respiratory symptoms from exposure to alkaline glutaraldehyde in medical services. Scand J Work Environ Health 1988;14:366-371.

40. Fowler JF Allergic contact dermatitis from glutaraldehyde exposure. J Occ Med 1989;31:852-3.

41. Norback D. Skin and respiratory symptoms from exposure to alkaline glutaraldehyde in medical services. Scand J Work Environ Health 1988;14:366-371.

42. Fisher AA. Reactions to glutaraldehyde with particular reference to radiologists and x-ray technicians. Cutis 1981;28:113- 122.

43. Norback D. Skin and respiratory symptoms from exposure to alkaline glutaraldehyde in medical services. Scand J Work Environ Health 1988;14:366- 371.

44. Jachuk SJ, Bound CL, Steel J, Blain PG. Occupational hazard in hospital staff exposed to 2 per cent glutaraldehyde in an endoscopy unit. J Soc Occup Med 1989;39:69-71.

45. Wiggins P, McCurdy SA, Zeidenberg W. Epistaxis due to glutaraldehyde exposure. J Occ Med 1989;31:854-857.

46. Corrado OJ, Osman J, Davies RJ. Asthma and rhinitis after exposure to glutaraldehyde in endoscopy units. Human Toxicol 1986;5:325-327.

47. Burge PS. Occupational risks of glutaraldehyde. Br Med J 1989;299:342.

48. Hathaway GJ, Proctor NH, Hughes JP, Fischman ML. Proctor and Hughes' chemical hazards of the workplace. (3rd ed.) New York: Van Nostrand Reinhold, 1991.

49. Norback D. Skin and respiratory symptoms from exposure to alkaline glutaraldehyde in medical services. Scand J Work Environ Health 1988;14:366-371.

50. Jachuk SJ, Bound CL, Steel J, Blain PG. Occupational hazard in hospital staff exposed to 2 per cent glutaraldehyde in an endoscopy unit. J Soc Occup Med 1989;39:69-71.

51. Leinster P, Baum JM, Baxter PJ. An assessment of exposure to glutaraldehyde in hospitals: typical exposure levels and recommended control measures. Br J Ind Med 1993;50:107-11.

52. Gestal JJ. Occupational hazards in hospitals: accidents, radiation, exposure to noxious chemicals, drug addiction and psychic problems, and assault. Br J Ind Med 1987;44:510-520.

53. IARC monographs, vol 36. Allyl compounds, aldehydes, epoxides and peroxides. Lyon: IARC, 1985.

54. Hathaway GJ, Proctor NH, Hughes JP, Fischman ML. Proctor and Hughes' chemical hazards of the workplace. (3rd ed.) New York: Van Nostrand Reinhold, 1991.

55. Bryant HE, Visser ND, Yoshida K. Ethylene oxide steriliser use and short term symptoms amongst workers. J Soc Occup Med 1989;39:101-106.

56. Deschamps D, Rosenberg N, Soler P, Maillard G, Fournier E, Salson D, Gervais P. Persistent asthma after accidental exposure to ethylene oxide. Br J Ind Med 1992;49:523-525.

57. Finelli P et al. Ethylene oxide- induced polyneuropathy: a clinical and electrophysiologic study. Arch Neurol 1983;40:419-421.

58. Kuzuhara S. Ethylene oxide polyneuropathy: report of 2 cases with biopsy studies of nerve and muscle. Clin Neurol 1982;22:707- 713.

59. Lynch DW, Lewis TR, Moorman WJ, et al. Carcinogenic and toxicologic effects of inhaled ethylene oxide and propylene oxide in F344 rats. Toxicol Appl Pharmacol 1984;76:69-84.

60. Hogstedt C, Aringer L, Gustavsson A. Epidemiologic support for ethylene oxide as a cancer-causing agent. JAMA 1986;255:1575-8.

61. Gardner MJ, Coggon D, Pannett B, Harris EC. Workers exposed to ethylene oxide: a follow up study. Br J Ind Med 1989;46:860- 865.

62. IARC monographs, suppl 7. 1987:205-207.

63. Elliott LJ, Ringenburg VL, Morelli-Schroth P, Halperin WE, Herrick RF. Ethylene oxide exposures in hospitals. Appl Ind Hyg 1988;3:141-145.

64. Elliott L, Mortimer V, Ringenberg V, Kercher S, O'Brien D. Effect of engineering controls and work practices in reducing ethylene-oxide exposure during the sterilisation of hospital supplies. Scand J Work Environ Health 1988;14(suppl 1):40-42.

65. Bryant HE, Visser ND, Yoshida K. Ethylene oxide steriliser use and short term symptoms amongst workers. J Soc Occup Med 1989;39:101-106.

66. Sass-Kortsak AM, Purdham JT, Bozek PR, Murphy JH. Exposure of hospital operating room personnel to potentially harmful environmental agents. Am Ind Hyg Assoc 1992;53:203-209.

67. Hathaway GJ, Proctor NH, Hughes JP, Fischman ML. Proctor and Hughes' chemical hazards of the workplace. (3rd ed.) New York: Van Nostrand Reinhold, 1991.

68. Blagodatin VM et al. Establishing the maximum permissible concentration of the methyl ester of methacrylic acid in the air of a work area. Gig Tr Prot Zabol 1976;6:508.

69. Seppalainen A, Rajaniemi R. Local neurotoxicity of methyl methacrylate among dental technicians. Am J Ind Med 1984;5:471-477.

70. Conde-Salazar L, Guimaraens D, Romero LV. Occupational allergic contact dermatitis from anaerobic acrylic sealants. Con Derm 1988;18:129-132.

71. Losewicz S et al. Occupational asthma due to methyl methacrylate and cyanoacrylates. Thorax 1985;40:8.

72. IARC monographs suppl 7. 1987:66.

73. Sass-Kortsak AM, Purdham JT, Bozek PR, Murphy JH. Exposure of hospital operating room personnel to potentially harmful environmental agents. Am Ind Hyg Assoc 1992;53:203-209.

74. Society of Radiographers. Preventing the darkroom disease: - health effects of toxic fumes produced in x-ray film processing. Society of Radiographers, 1991.

75. Industrial Injuries Advisory Council. Occupational Asthma. (Cmnd 1244). London: HMSO, 1990.

76. Norrpa H, Sorsa M, Vaino H, et al. Increased sister chromatid exchanges frequencies in lymphocytes of nurses handling cytostatic drugs. Scand J Work Env Health 1980;6:229.

CHAPTER 4

1. Commission on the Provision of Surgical Services. Report of the working party on guidelines for day care surgery. London: Royal College of Surgeons of England, 1992.

2. Steven IM, A scavenging system for use in paediatric anaesthesia. Anaesthesia & Intensive Care. 1990;18(2):238-40.

3. Logan M, Farmer JG. Anaesthesia and the ozone layer. Br J Anaes 1989;63:645-647.

4. Westhope R and Blutstein H. Anaesthetic agents and the ozone layer. Anaesth & Intensive Care 1990;18(1):102-4.

5. Radke J, Fabian P. The ozone layer and its modification by N20 and inhalation anaesthetics. Anaesthetist 1991;40(8):429-33.

6. HSE. Occupational exposure limits EH40-1994. London: HMSO, 1994.

7. Davenport HT, Halsey MJ, Wardley-Smith B, Wright BM. Measurement and reduction of occupational exposure to inhaled anaesthetics. Br Med J 1976;2:1219-1221.

8. Thompson JM, Sithamparanadarajah R, Hutton P, Robinson JS, Stephen WI. Evaluation of the efficacy of an active scavenger for controlling air contamination in an operating theatre. Br J Anaesth 1981;53:235- 240.

9. Davenport HT, Halsey MJ, Wardley-Smith B, Wright BM. Measurement and reduction of occupational exposure to inhaled anaesthetics. Br Med J 1976;2:1219-1221.

10. Davenport HT, Halsey MJ et al. Occupational exposure to anaesthetics in 20 hospitals. Anaesthesia 1980;35(4):354-9.

11. Thompson JM, Sithamparanadarajah R, Hutton P, Robinson JS, Stephen WI. Evaluation of the efficacy of an active scavenger for controlling air contamination in an operating theatre. Br J Anaesth 1981;53:235- 240.

12. Boyland PC. Gas scavenging at Queen Elizabeth II Hospital, Portsmouth. Hospital Engineering Feb 1982:13-16.

13. Thompson JM, Sithamparanadarajah R, Robinson JS, Stephen WI. Occupational exposure to nitrous oxide, halothane and isopropanol in operating theatres. Health and Hygiene 1987;8:60-68.

14. Gray WM. Occupational exposure to nitrous oxide in four hospitals. Anaesthesia 1989;44:511-514.

15. Gardner RJ. Inhalation anaesthetics - exposure control : A statistical comparison of personal exposures in operating theatres with and without anaesthetic gas scavenging. Ann Occup Hyg 1989;33:159-173.

16. Rajhans GS, Brown DA, Whaley D, Wong L, Guirevis SS. Hygiene aspects of occupational exposure to waste anaesthetic gases in ontario hospitals. Ann Occup Hyg 1989;33:27-45.

17. Sass-Kortsak AM, Purdham JT, Bozek PR, Murphy JH. Exposure of hospital operating room personnel to potentially harmful environmental agents. Am Ind Hyg Assoc 1992;53:203- 209.

18. Thompson JM, Sithamparanadarajah R, Robinson JS, Stephen WI. Occupational exposure to nitrous oxide, halothane and isopropanol in operating theatres. Health and Hygiene 1987;8:60-68.

19. Gray WM. Occupational exposure to nitrous oxide in four hospitals. Anaesthesia 1989;44:511-514.

20. Gardner RJ. Inhalation anaesthetics - exposure control : A statistical comparison of personal exposures in operating theatres with and without anaesthetic gas scavenging. Ann Occup Hyg 1989;33:159-173.

21. Rajhans GS, Brown DA, Whaley D, Wong L, Guirevis SS. Hygiene aspects of occupational exposure to waste anaesthetic gases in ontario hospitals. Ann Occup Hyg 1989;33:27-45.

33. The Ionising Radiations Regulations 1985. SI 1333. London: HMSO, 1985.

34. The Medicines (Administration of radioactive substances) Regulations 1978. SI 1006. London: HMSO, 1978.

35. Tobias J. What went wrong at Exeter. Br Med J 1988;297:372-73.

36. Kam KC. The precautions necessary for handling sealed and unsealed radioactive sources. In: Wootton R, ed. Radiation protection of patients. Cambridge: Cambridge University Press, 1993.

37. Hughes JS and O'Riordon MC. Radiation exposure of the UK population - 1993 review, NRPB-R263. London: HMSO, 1993.

38. Mountford PJ, O'Doherty MJ, Forge NI, Jeffries A, Coakley AJ. Radiation dose rates from adult patients undergoing nuclear medicine investigations. Nucl Med Commun 1991;12(9):767-77.

39. HSC. Approved Code of Practice. The protection of persons against ionising radiation arising from any work activity. London: HMSO, 1985.

40. Wootton R. Radiation protection of patients. Cambridge: Cambridge University Press, 1993.

41. National Radiological Protection Board. Living with radiation. London: HMSO, 1991.

42. HSE policy statement on radiation protection in the UK. Health and Safety Commission 1993.

43. Documents of the NRPB, issue 2, volume 4:1-82. 1993.

44. The Ionising Radiations Regulations 1985. SI 1333. London: HMSO, 1985.

CHAPTER 6

1. Haley RW, Culver DH, White JW et al. The efficacy of infection surveillance and control programs in preventing nosocomial infections in university hospitals. Am J Epidemiol 1985;121:182-205.

2. Health and Safety Advisory Committee. Safe working and the prevention of infection in the mortuary and post-mortem room. London: HMSO, 1991.

3. Department of Health. Mortuary and post-mortem room, Health Building Note 20. London: HMSO, 1991.

4. Lucas S B. HIV and necropsy. J Clin Pathol 1993;46:1071-1075.

5. Health Services Advisory Committee. Safe working and the prevention of infection in the mortuary and post-mortem room. London: HMSO, 1991.

6. Centres for Disease Control. Nosocomial transmission of multi-drug-resistant tuberculosis among HIV infected persons - Florida and New York, 1988-1991. MMWR 1991;40:585-91.

7. Centres for Disease Control. Nosocomial transmission of multi-drug resistant tuberculosis to health-care workers and HIV infected patients in an urban hospital - Florida. MMWR 1990;39:718-22.

8. Di Perri G, Cruciani M, Danzi MC, Luzzati R, Chcchiu GD, Malena M, et al. Nosocomial epidemic of active tuberculosis among HIV-infected patients. Lancet 1989;334:1502-4.

9. Nardell EA. Nosocomial tuberculosis in the AIDS era. Strategies for interupting transmission in developing countries. Bull Int Union Tuberc Lung Dis 1991;66(2-3):107-11.

10. Watson JM. Tuberculosis in Britain today. BMJ 1993;306:221-2.

11. Pozniak A, Watson JM. Nosocomial transmission of tuberculosis in AIDS care centres. Communicable Disease Report 1992;2:R40-2.

12. Hovig B. Lower respiratory tract infections associated with respiratory therapy and anaesthetic equipment. J Hospital Infect 1981;2:301-5.

13. Cefai C, Richards J, Gould KF, McPeake P. An outbreak of Acinetobacter respiratory tract infection resulting form incomplete disinfection of ventilatory equipment. J Hospital Med 1990;15:177-82.

14. Levin AS, Caiaffa Filho HH, Sinto SI, Sabbaga E, Barone AA. An outbreak of nosocomial Legionnaires' disease in a renal transplant unit in Sao Paulo, Brazil. Legionellosis Study Team. J Hosp Infect 1991;18:243.

15. Hanson PJV, Jeffries DJ, Batten JC, Collins JV. Infection control revisited: dilemma facing today's bronchoscopists. Br Med J 1988;297:185-87.

16. Birnie GG, Quigley EM, Clements GB, et al. Endoscopic transmission of hepatitis B virus. Gut 1983;24:171-174.

17. Webb F, Vall-Spinosa A. Outbreak of Serratia marcescence associated with the flexible fibrebronchoscope. Chest 1975;68:703-8.

18. Siegman-Igra Y, Inbar G, Campus A. An outbreak of pulmonary pseudo-infection by Serratia marcescence. J Hosp Infect 1985;6:218-20.

19. Pappas SA, Schaaff DM, DiConstanzo MB, King FW, Sharp JT. Contamination of flexible bronchoscopes. Am Rev Respir Dis 1983;127:391-2.

20. Hanson PJV, Jeffries DJ, Batten JC, Collins JV. Infection control revisited: dilemma facing today's bronchoscopists. Br Med J 1988;297:185-87.

21. British Society of Gastroenterology. Cleaning and disinfection of equipment for gastrointestinal flexible endoscopy: interim recommendations of a Working Party. Gut 1988;29:1134-51.

22. Douvin C, Simon D, Zinelabidine H, Wirquin V, Perlemuter L, Dheaumeux D. An outbreak of hepatitis B in an endocrinology unit traced to a capillary-blood-sampling device. N Eng J Med 1990;322:57-8.

23. Cartwright K, Turner H. Safety aspects of outstationed laboratory equipment. J Hospital Infect 1992;20:225-31.

24. Oakley K, Gooch C, Cockcroft A. Review of management of incidents involving exposure to blood in a London teaching hospital, 1989-91. BMJ 1992;304:949-51.

25. Astbury C, Baxter PJ. Infection risks in hospital staff from blood : Hazardous injury rates and acceptance of hepatitis B immunisation. J Soc Occ Med 1990;40:92-3.

26. Richmond PW, McCabe M, Davies JP, Thomas DM. Perforation of gloves in an accident and emergency department. BMJ 1992;304:879-80.

27. Hussain SA, Latif ABA, Choudray AA. Risk to surgeons: A survey of accidental injuries during operations. Br J Surg 1988;75:314-6.

28. Brough SF, Hunt TM, Barrie WW. Surgical glove perforations. Br J Surg 1988;75:317.

29. Matta H, Thompson AM, Rainey JB. Does wearing two pairs of gloves protect operating theatre staff from skin contamination? Br Med J 1988;297:597-8.

30. Shpuntoff H, Shpuntoff RL. High- speed dental handpieces and spread of airborne infections. NY State Dental J 1993;59:21- 3.

31. British Medical Association. A code of practice for the safe use and disposal of sharps. London: BMA, 1990.

32. Heap D. Health care industry. Occ Med 1993;43:47-50.

33. Department of Health. Protecting health care workers and patients from hepatitis B. Recommendations of the Advisory Group on hepatitis. London: Department of Health, 1993.

34. Besso L, Rovere A, Peano G, Menardi G, Fenoglio LM, Fenoglio S, Ghezzi PM. Prevalence of HCV antibodies in a Uraemic population undergoing maintenance dialysis therapy and in staff members of the dialysis unit. Nephron 1992;61:304.

35. Petrarulo F, Maggi P, Sacchetti A, Pallotta G, Dagostino F, Basile C. HCV infection occupational hazard of dialysis units and virus spread among relatives of dialysed patients. Nephron 1992;61:302.

36. Kiyosawa K, Sodeyama T, Tanaka E, et al. Hepatitis C in hospital employees with needlestick injuries. Ann Intern Med 1991;115:367-9.

37. Heptonstall J, Gill ON, Porter K, Black MB, Gilbart VL. Health care workers and HIV; surveillance of occupationally acquired infection in the United Kingdom. Communicable Disease Report 1993;3:R147-R152.

38. UK Health Departments. HIV/AIDS - Infected health care wokers : guidance on the management of infected health care workers. Recommendations of the expert advisory group on AIDS. London: DoH, 1994.

39. Matthews WB. Bovine spongiform encephalopathy. BMJ 1990;300:412.

40. Brown P. Human growth hormone therapy and Creutzfeldt-Jakob Disease: A drama in three acts. Paediatrics 1988;81:85-92.

41. Miller DC. Creutzfeldt-Jakob Disease in histopathology technicians. NEJM 1988;318:853.

CHAPTER 7

1. Collins CH, Kennedy DA. The treatment and disposal of clinical waste. HHSC Handbook. Leeds: H & H Scientific Consultants, 1993.

2. British Medical Association. Hazardous waste and human health. Oxford: OUP, 1991.

3. HSC. The safe disposal of clinical waste. London: Health and Safety Commission, 1982.

4. BS 3316: 1987. A code of practice for the design, specification, installation and commissioning of incinerators or the destruction of hospital waste. London: British Standards Institution, 1987.

5. Department of the Environment. The Government's reply to the second report from the environment committee, toxic waste. (Cmnd 679). London: HMSO, 1989.

6. Controlled Waste (Registration of Carriers and Seizure of Vehicles) Regulations 1992. SI 588. London: HMSO, 1992.

7. Environmental Protection Act (Duty of Care) Regulations 1991. SI 2839. London: HMSO, 1991.

8. HSC. Safe Disposal of Clinical Waste. London: Health and Safety Commission, 1992.

9. British Medical Association. A code of practice for the safe use and disposal of sharps. London: BMA, 1990.

10. Kiyosawa K, Sodeyama T, Tanaka E, et al. Hepatitis C in hospital employees with needlestick injuries. Ann Intern Med 1991;115:367-9.

11. CDC. Acquired immunodeficiency syndrome (AIDS). Precautions for health care workers and allied professionals. MMWR 1983;32:450-51.

12. British Medical Association. A code of practice for the safe use and disposal of sharps. London: BMA, 1990.

13. HSC. The Safe Disposal of Clinical Waste. London: Health and Safety Commission, 1982.

14. Department of Health. Specification for containers for sharps. London: DoH, 1990.

15. HSC. The Safe Disposal of Clinical Waste. London: Health and Safety Commission, 1992.

16. Deparment of the Environment. Waste Management Paper No 25: Clinical Waste. London: DoE, 1983.

17. London Waste Regulation Authority. Clinical Waste - an Appraisal. London: LWRA, 1989.

18. London Waste Regulation Authority. Guidelines for the segregation, handling and transport of clinical waste. London: LWRA, 1989.

19. The management of clinical waste. London: National Association of Waste Disposal Contractors, 1991.

20. Air pollution from crown property. A report. Brighton: National Association for Clean Air, 1991.

21. Peterson ML. Pathogens associated with solid waste processing. Washington: US Environmental Protection Agency, SW-49r, Government Printing Office, 1971.

22. BS 3316: 1987. A code of practice for the design, specification, installation and commissioning of incinerators or the destruction of hospital waste. London: British Standards Institution, 1987.

23. HM Inspectorate of Pollution. Chemical waste incineration, revised note on best practical means. London: HMSO, 1989.

24. Council Directive on the reduction of air pollution from existing municipal waste incineration plants. 89/429/EEC.

25. Secretary of State's Guidance Note PG5/1. Clinical waste incineration processes under 1 tonne per hour. London: HMSO, 1991.

26. Chief Inspector's Guidance to Inspectors: Waste disposal and recycling. Clinical waste. HMIP Process Guidance Note IPR 5/2. London: HMSO, 1992.

27. BS 3316: 1987. A code of practice for the design, specification, installation and commissioning of incinerators or the destruction of hospital waste. London: British Standards Institution, 1987.

28. HM Inspectorate of Pollution. Chemical waste incineration, revised note on best practical means. London: HMSO, 1989.

29. Council Directive on the reduction of air pollution from existing municipal waste incineration plants. 89/429/EEC.

30. Secretary of State's Guidance Note PG5/1. Clinical waste incineration processes under 1 tonne per hour. London: HMSO, 1991.

31. Chief Inspector's Guidance to Inspectors: Waste disposal and recycling. Clinical Waste. HMIP Process Guidance Note IPR 5/2. London: HMSO, 1992.

32. London Waste Regulation Authority. Clinical waste - an appraisal. London: LWRA, 1989.

33. London Waste Regulation Authority. Guidelines for the segregation, handling and transport of clinical waste. London: LWRA, 1989.

34. Institute of Environmental Health Officers. Survey - incinerators. London: IEHO, 1992.

35. Draft Council Directive on Landfill. 91/C 130/01/EEC.

36. London Waste Regulation Authority. Clinical waste - an appraisal. London: LWRA, 1989.

37. London Waste Regulation Authority. Guidelines for the segregation, handling and transport of clinical waste. London: LWRA, 1989.

38. Draft Council Directive on Landfill. 91/C 130/01/EEC.

39. British Medical Association. Hazardous waste and human health. Oxford: OUP, 1991.

40. Collins CH. Laboratory acquired infections. (2nd ed.) Oxford: Butterworth-Heinemann, 1988.

41. Collins CH, Lyne PM, Grange JM. eds. Collins and Lyne's microbiological methods. (6th ed.) Oxford: Butterworth-Heinemann, 1989.

42. Advisory Committee on Dangerous Pathogens. Categorization of pathogens according to hazard and categories of containment. London: HMSO, 1990.

43. Health Services Advisory Committee. Safe working and the prevention of infection in clinical laboratories. London: HMSO, 1991.

44. Health Services Advisory Committee. Safe disposal of clinical waste. London: HMSO, 1982, revised 1992.

45. Daschner FD. Infectious waste management - will science, common sense and cost benefit prevail?. Infect Control Hosp Epidemiol 1989;10:440-41.

46. US EPA. Guide to pollution control. selected waste streams. US EPA/627/7-90/009. Cincinnati: Center for Environmental Research Information, 1990.

47. Commission of the European Communities. Analysis of priority waste streams health care waste, Information Document Summary. December 1993.

CHAPTER 8

1. British Medical Association. Our genetic future. Oxford: OUP, 1992.

2. Ellis CJ, Katifi H, Weller RO. A further British case of growth hormone induced Creutzfeld-Jacob disease. J Neurol Neurosurg Psychiatry 1992;55(12):1200-2.

3. Lazorush. Suspension of the Australian human pituitary hormone programme. Med J Aust 143(2):57-9.

4. British Medical Association. Our genetic future. Oxford: OUP, 1992.

5. Sleigh JD. Escherichia Coli: Klebsiella: Proteus: Providencia. In: Mackie and McCartney, Medical Microbiology. Eds Duguid JP, Marmion BP, Swain RHA. London: Churchill Livingstone, 1978: 327-333.

6. British Medical Association. Our genetic future. Oxford: OUP, 1992.

7. Wright G, Carver A, Cottom D, Reeves D, Scott A, Simons P, Wilmut I, Garner I, Colman A. High level of expression of active human alpha-1-antitrypsin in the milk of transgenic sheep. Biotechnology 1991;9:830-4.

8. Janne J, Hyttinen JM, Peura T, Tolvanen M, Alhonen L, Halmekyto M. Transgenic animals as bioproducers of therapeutic proteins. Department of Biochemistry & Biotechnology, University of Kuopio, Finland. Annals of Medicine 1992;24(4):273-80.

9. British Medical Association. Our genetic future. Oxford: OUP, 1992.

10. British Medical Association. Medical ethics today: Its practice and philosophy. London: BMJ Publishing Group, 1993.

11. Health and Safety (Genetic manipulation) Regulations 1978. SI 752. London: HMSO, 1978.

12. Genetic Manipulation Regulations 1989. SI 1810. London: HMSO, 1989.

13. Control of Substances Hazardous to Health Regulations 1988. SI 1657. London: HMSO, 1988.

14. The Genetically Modified Organisms (Contained use) Regulations, 1992. SI 3217. HMSO, 1992.

15. News. Error of judgement over gene safety rules. Nature 1994;367:499.

16. Health and Safety Executive. Guide to Genetically Modified Organisms (Contained Use) Regulations HSE, 1993

17. DoH Press Release, H93/767.

18. British Medical Association. Medical ethics today: its practice and philosophy. London: BMJ Publishing Group, 1993.

CHAPTER 9

1. TUC. The deregulation and contracting out Bill: Health and Safety: Background brief. January 1994.

2. National Audit Office. Enforcing Health and Safety Legislation in the Workplace. Report by the Comptroller and Auditor General. London: HMSO 208, 1994.

3. Health and Safety Executive. Successful Health and Safety Management: Health and Safety Services booklet HS(G)65. London: HMSO, 1991.

4. Council Directive on the introduction of measures to encourage improvements in the health and safety at work of pregnant workers and workers who have recently given birth or are breastfeeding (tenth individual Directive within the meaning of Article 16 (1) of Directive 89/391/EEC). 92/85/EEC.

5. Makin PJ, Rout U, Cooper CL. Job satisfaction and occupational stress among general practitioners - a pilot study. JR Coll Gen Pract 1988;38:303-6.

6. British Medical Association. Stress and the Medical Profession. London: BMA, 1992.

7. Faculty of Occupational Medicine. Report of the Faculty of Occupational Medicine's Working Party on environmental medicine. London: FOM, 1993.

8. Department of Health. Managing the New NHS: Proposal to determine new NHS regions and establish new Regional Health Authorities. Consultation Document. London: DoH, 1 November 1993.

9. ibid.

10. Department of Health. White Paper, The Health of the Nation: A Strategy for Health in England. (Cmnd 1986). London: HMSO, 1992.

11. Cooke RA, Hodgson ES. General Practitioners and Health and Safety at Work. BMJ 1992;305:1044.

12. Faculty of Occupational Medicine. Report of the Faculty of Occupational Medicine's Working Party on environmental medicine. London: FOM, 1993.

13. Harrington JM and Gill FS. Occupational Health. (3rd ed.) Oxford: Blackwell Scientific Publications, 1993.

CHAPTER 10

1. Atkin K, Lunt N, Parker G, Hirst M. Nurses count: a national census of practice nurses. Social Policy Research Unit, University of York, 1993.
2. Department of Health. Managing the New NHS: Proposal to determine new NHS regions and establish new Regional Health Authorities. Consultation Document. London: DoH, 1 November 1993
3. Ellis N. Employing staff. (5th ed.) London: BMJ Publishing Group, 1994.
4. Health and Safety Executive, Medical aspects of occupational asthma, Guidance Note MS25. London: HMSO, 1991.
5. London Waste Regulation Authority, Annual Report 1992/93. London: LWRA, 1994.
6. British Medical Association. A code of practice for sterilisation of instruments and control of cross infection. London: BMA, 1989.
7. British Medical Association. A code of practice for the safe use and disposal of sharps. London: BMA, 1990.
8. NHS (General Medical Services) Regulations 1992, Statement of Fees and Allowances.
9. NHS Estates. Health Building Note 46. General medical practice premises for the provision of primary health care services. London: HMSO, 1991.

CHAPTER 11

1. Health and Safety at Work Act 1974. London: HMSO, 1974.
2. Control of Substances Hazardous to Health Regulations 1988. SI 1657. London: HMSO, 1988.
3. Workplace (Health, Safety and Welfare) Regulations 1992. SI 3004. London: HMSO, 1992.
4. Environmental Protection Act 1990. London: HMSO, 1990.
5. The Ionising Radiation Regulations 1985. SI 1333. London: HMSO, 1985.
6. Advisory Committee on Dangerous Pathogens. Categorisation of pathogens according to hazard and categories of containment. (2nd ed.) London: HMSO, 1990.
7. NHS Executive, Risk Management in the NHS. London: DoH, 1993.

8. Society of Radiographers. Preventing the darkroom disease:- Health effects of toxic fumes produced in x-ray film processing. London: Society of Radiographers, 1991.

9. BS 6834. Specification for active anaesthetic gas scavenging systems. London: British Standards Institution, 1987.

10. NHS Estates. Health Building Note 26, Operating Department. London: HMSO, 1991.

11. BS 7258. Laboratory fume cupboards. London: British Standards Institution, 1990.

12. Advisory Committee on Dangerous Pathogens,. Categorisation of pathogens according to hazard and categories of containment. (2nd ed.) London: HMSO, 1990.

13. Health Technical Memorandum (HTM) 2040. The control of legionellae in health care premises - a code of practice. London: HMSO, 1993.

14. Public Health Laboratory Service. New code of practice for the control of legionellas in health care premises. Communicable Disease Report Weekly 1994:4(5);1.

15. Health and Safety Executive. Manual Handling Operations Regulations 1992. Guidance on Regulations. London: HMSO, 1992.

16. Health and Safety Executive. Display Screen Equipment Work (Health and Safety Display Screen Equipment) Regulations 1992. Guidance on Regulations. London: HMSO, 1992.

17. Department of Environment. Sustainable development: the UK strategy. (Cmnd 2426). London: HMSO, 1994

18. NHS Estates. Towards a Healthier Estate. Annual Report 1991-92. London: Department of Health, Central Office of Information, 1992.

19. National Association of Health Authorities and Trusts. Day surgery: Report by the day surgery task force. Birmingham: NAHAT, 1993.

20. Department of the Environment. Improving environmental quality, The Government's proposals for a new, independent environment agency. London: DoE, 1991.

21. Department of Environment. Sustainable development: the UK strategy. (Cmnd 2426). London: HMSO, 1994

22. Royal College of Nursing. 50 steps towards a healthy environment. London: RCN, 1992.

CHAPTER 12

1. Health and Safety Executive. Successful Health and Safety Management: Health and Safety Services booklet HS(G)65. London: HMSO, 1991.

2. Heptonstall J, Gill ON, Porter K, Black MB, Gilbart VL. Health care workers and HIV; surveillance of occupationally acquired infection in the United Kingdom. Communicable Disease Report 1993:3;R147-R152.

3. Chant K, Lowe D, Rubin G, Manning W et al. Patient-to-patient transmission of HIV in private surgical consulting rooms. Lancet 1993; 342:1548-9.

4. BMJ News. Australians investigate hepatitis C cases. BMJ 1994;308: 1256-7.

5. British Medical Association. Stress and the medical profession. London: BMA, 1992.

6. Symington I S. Occupational medicine in the National Health Service. Postgrad Med J 1992;68:663-670.

7. British Medical Association. Hazardous waste and human health. Oxford: OUP, 1991.

8. Department of Health. Managing the New NHS: Proposal to determine new NHS regions and establish new Regional Health Authorities. Consultation Document. London: DoH, 1 November 1993.

9. Public Health : responsibilities of the NHS and the roles of others. Advice of the committee set up to undertake a review of HC(88)64. 1993.

10. National Audit Office. Enforcing Health and Safety Legislation in the Workplace. Report by the Comptroller and Auditor General. London: HMSO, 1994.

11. TUC. The deregulation and contracting out Bill: Health and Safety: Background brief. January 1994

12. National Audit Office. Enforcing Health and Safety Legislation in the Workplace. Report by the Comptroller and Auditor General. London: HMSO, 1994.

13. British Medical Association. The morbidity and mortality of the medical profession. London: BMA, 1993.

14. Health and Safety Executive. Your patients and their work: An introduction to occupational health for family doctors. London: HSE, 1992.

15. Centres for Disease Control. Nosocomial transmission of multi-drug-resistant tuberculosis among HIV infected persons - Florida and New York, 1988-1991. MMWR 1991;40:585-91.

16. Centres for Disease Control. Nosocomial transmission of multi-drug resistant tuberculosis to health-care workers and HIV infected patients in an urban hospital - Florida. MMWR 1990;39:718-22.

17. Di Perri G, Cruciani M, Danzi MC, Luzzati R, Chcchiu GD, Malena M, et al. Nosocomial epidemic of active tuberculosis among HIV-infected patients. Lancet 1989;334:1502-4.

18. Watson JM. Tuberculosis in Britain today. BMJ 1993;306:221-2.

19. British Medical Association. A code of practice for the safe use and disposal of sharps. London: BMA, 1990.

20. British Medical Association. A code of practice for sterilisation of instruments and control of cross infection. London: BMA, 1989.

21. Department of Health. Guidance for clinical health workers: protection against infection with HIV and hepatitis viruses. Recommendations of the experts advisory group on AIDS. London: HMSO, 1990.

22. Health and Safety Executive. Needlestick Injuries. HSE Information Sheet. London: HSE, 1993.

23. British Medical Association. Immunisation against hepatitis B. London: BMA, 1987.

24. British Medical Association. Hazardous waste and human health. London: BMA, 1991.

25. Department of the Environment. Waste Management paper No 25: Clinical Waste. London: DoE, 1983.

26. British Medical Association. A code of practice for the safe use and disposal of sharps. London: BMA, 1990.

27. British Medical Association. A code of practice for sterilisation of instruments and control of cross infection. London: BMA, 1989.

28. Managing the New NHS, Proposal to determine new NHS regions and establish new Regional Health Authorities, Consultation Document. London: DoH, 1 November, 1993.

29. Department of Health. Managing the New NHS: Proposal to determine new NHS regions and establish new Regional Health Authorities. Consultation Document. London: DoH, 1 November 1993.

Index